Ulcerative Colitis

Editor

Colm A. O'Morain, M.D., M.Sc., F.R.C.P.I.

Consultant Gastroenterologist
Department of Gastroenterology
Meath/Adelaide Hospitals
Dublin, Ireland
and
Senior Lecturer in Gastroenterology
Director of Clinical Studies
Trinity College
Dublin, Ireland

CRC Press
Boca Raton   Ann Arbor   Boston

Library of Congress Cataloging-in-Publication Data

Ulcerative colitis/editor, Colm A. O'Morain.
      p.   cm.
    Includes bibliographical references.
    Includes index.
    ISBN 0-8493-5498-6
    1. Ulcerative colitis.   I. O'Morain, Colm A.
    [DNLM: 1. Colitis, Ulcerative. 2. Inflammatory Bowel Diseases.   WI
522 U361]
RC862.C63U43   1991
616.3'447--dc20
DNLM/DLC
for Library of Congress   90-2607
                                                   CIP

Direct all inquiries to CRC Press, Inc., 2000 Corporate Blvd., N.W., Boca Raton, Florida 33431.

© 1991 by CRC Press, Inc.

International Standard Book Number 0-8493-5498-6

Library of Congress Card Number 90-2607
Printed in the United States

PREFACE

Ulcerative colitis remains one of the greatest challenges in medicine today. It is usually classified with Crohn's disease and the two are collectively called inflammatory bowel disease. There is considerable overlap between the two conditions suggesting a common etiology or perhaps the spectrum of one disease. There are clear-cut differences in most cases to allow a confident diagnosis to be made. In this book the main subject matter is ulcerative colitis. I feel that inflammatory bowel disease should be considered as at least two diseases. Further progress and knowledge of the cause of these diseases will occur if the disease is split rather than lumped together. Ulcerative colitis is characterized by inflammation confined to part or the whole of the colon. It almost always begins in the rectum and extends proximally.

In active disease the lamina propria is infiltrated by polymorphonuclear leukocytes, lymphocytes, and macrophages. With severe inflammation the crypts may be distended with polymorphonuclear leukocytes to form crypt abscesses. These may rupture to form microscopic ulcers. Other features include goblet cell depletion and glandular destruction. It is a disease characterized by relapses and remissions. It frequently affects young people. The symptoms are distressing, with diarrhea frequently mixed with blood as the predominant symptom during relapse. Diagnosis is usually made by colonoscopy and biopsy. Corticosteroids are used to treat the acute attack, and sulfasalazine and the more developed salicylates have been shown to lower the rate of relapse. Surgery has an important role in the management. Indications for surgical resection are failure of medical treatment of acute attacks or extensive disease with chronic symptoms. Emergency colectomy may have to be performed in the presence of perforation or toxic megacolon in a patient with a severe attack of the disease.

There is genetic predisposition to the disease. Differential diagnosis includes the irritable bowel syndrome and specific forms of inflammatory gastrointestinal disorders. The most common would be due to infectious agents which may give a clinical and pathological picture indistinguishable from inflammatory bowel disease. Specific infections include those caused by bacteria (*Campylobacter, Salmonella, Shigella, Yersinia,* mycobacteria), entamoeba, histocytic viruses, cytomegalovirus, fungi, and histoplasma. Other diseases with similar presentations are ischemic colitis, radiation colitis, diverticulitis, and large bowel neoplasm.

The etiology of ulcerative colitis is unknown. Various theories have been proposed including infectious, immunologic, dietary, and psychological. A variety of humoral and cell-mediated abnormalities have been detected in the peripheral circulation and intestine, suggesting that immune phenomenon are involved in the pathogenesis of the disease, but it is not clear whether they are a primary or secondary phenomenon. Similarly, in the case of psychological factors, it is not certain that the characteristic personality associated with ulcerative colitis could be a consequence of a chronic disease.

Inflammation and inflammatory products are important in the pathogenesis of ulcerative colitis. Polymorphonuclear leukocytes are prominent in the inflamed mucosa in ulcerative colitis. Enzymes released from the cells would contribute to the inflammatory process. Arachidonic acid is released from cellular phospholipids by the activity of various phospholipases. It is subsequently metabolized either through the cyclooxygenase pathway to prostaglandins (PGs), prostacyclins (PG1$_2$), and thrombuxuas (TXs) or through the lipoxygenase pathway to hydroxyperoxyeicosatetranoic acid (HPETES), hydroxyeicosatetranoic acid (HETES), and leukotrienes (LT). These products play a central role in inflammatory responses. *In vitro* experiments show that colonic mucosal biopsies for patients with active ulcerative colitis have high concentrations of PGE$_2$, LTB$_4$, and 5HETE compared to normal tissues which fall when the disease remits.

Treatment with drugs, steroids, and sulfasalazine may exert its therapeutic effect by inhibiting prostaglandin synthesis. In addition, products of arachidonic acid and its metabolite have a significant role in immune regulation. PGE_2 has been shown to stimulate suppression cell activity and LTB_4 is a potent chemotactic activity and may play a central role in mediation of interleukin 2 helper signals for interferon gamma production.

Intestinal epithelial cells provide a physical barrier separating luminal antigens and pathogens from the lamina propria. An abnormal mucus layer could be another manifestation of deficient epithelial cell function. A negative correlation with smoking has been described in that ulcerative colitis patients are more likely to be nonsmokers. It is possible that smoking could exert its effect by enhancing mucus production.

From this introduction it is obvious that the study of ulcerative colitis requires a multidisciplinary approach. I have been involved in inflammatory bowel disease research for over 10 years. In 1988 I was an author of a book on Crohn's disease. I thought it would be appropriate that I should edit a book on ulcerative colitis. For this book I have asked leading world experts, with whom I have met and collaborated over the years, to contribute. I have been impressed with their work and dedication to the study of this disease and hope this book will give the flavor of the multifacets of this disease and encourage further work to elucidate the cause and the search for more effective treatment.

THE EDITOR

Colm A. O'Morain is a Consultant Gastroenterologist at the Meath and Adelaide Hospitals, Dublin, Ireland, and Senior Lecturer in Gastroenterology and Director of Clinical Studies at Trinity College, Dublin.

He received his M.B. BCh. B.A.O. degree from the University College, Dublin, in 1972; completed his internship and residency at the Mater Hospital, Dublin; and was a Visiting Fellow in Gastroenterology at Centre Hepato. Gastroenterologie in Nice, France, in 1975. He obtained membership in the Royal College of Physicians of Ireland in 1977, Master of Science in Biochemistry from the University of London, 1980, M.D. thesis from the National University of Ireland, 1982, and Diploma in Immunology from the University of London, 1983.

Dr. O'Morain was Senior Registrar and a Medical Research Council Fellow in Gastroenterology at Northwick Park Hospital and Clinical Research Centre, London, and the Royal Postgraduate Medical School, Hammersmith, London, from 1978 to 1983. He was a Fogarty Fellow at the Albert Einstein College of Medicine, New York, from 1983 to 1985.

Dr. O'Morain is Chairman of the Division of Medicine and Director of Undergraduate Studies at the Meath, Adelaide, and National Children's Hospitals, Dublin; a Council Member of the Royal College of Physicians of Ireland, and a Fellow of the Royal College of Physicians of Ireland. He is the Secretary of the Irish Society of Gastroenterology and is President of the Academh Na Lianna, the Irish Speaking Doctors Association. He is also a member of the British Society of Gastroenterology and the American Gastroenterology Association.

The recipient of many research grants, Dr. O'Morain's main research interest for the past 10 years has been inflammatory bowel disease, and he has published widely on this subject.

CONTRIBUTORS

Anthony Thomas Roger Axon, M.B., M.D., F.R.C.P.
Consultant Physician
Department of Gastroenterology
Leeds General Infirmary
Leeds, England

Nigel K. Boughton-Smith, M.Sc., Ph.D.
Senior Scientist
Department of Pharmacology
Wellcome Research Laboratories
Beckenham, England

Denis Anthony Burke, M.B., M.R.C.P.
Senior Registrar
Department of Gastroenterology
Freeman Hospital
Newcastle upon Tyne, England

Graham Francis Cope, M.I.Biol., Ph.D.
Research Fellow
Department of Medicine
St. James' University Hospital
Leeds, England

Michael G. Courtney, M.B., M.R.C.P.I.
Senior Registrar
Department of Gastroenterology
St. Thomas' Hospital
London, England

Kiron M. Das, M.D., Ph.D.
Professor of Medicine, Microbiology, and
  Molecular Genetics
Department of Medicine
UMDNJ-Robert Wood Johnson Medical
  School
New Brunswick, New Jersey

Jay A. Gates, M.D.
Postdoctoral Fellow in Gastrointestinal
  Pathology
Department of Pathology
Yale University School of Medicine
New Haven, Connecticut

Sylvia Gyde, M.A., B.M., B.Ch.Oxon., M.F.C.M. Law
Director of Public Health
North Birmingham Health Authority
Erdington, Birmingham, England

Richard V. Heatley, M.D.
Consultant Physician
Department of Medicine
St. James' University Hospital
Leeds, England

Francis B. V. Keane, M.D., F.R.C.S.
Department of Surgery
Adelaide Hospital and
Consultant Surgeon/Senior Lecturer
Trinity College
Dublin, Ireland

Dermot Kelleher, M.B., M.R.C.P.I.
Lecturer
Department of Clinical Medicine
Trinity College and
Honorary Senior Registrar
Department of Gastroenterology
St. James' Hospital
Dublin, Ireland

Jerry Kelleher, Ph.D.
Senior Lecturer
Department of Medicine
St. James' University Hospital
Leeds, England

John Francis Mayberry, M.D., F.R.C.P.I.
Consultant Physician
Department of Medicine
Leicester General Hospital
Leicester, England

Thérèse McCall, Ph.D.
Research Scientist
Department of Pharmacology
Wellcome Research Laboratories
Beckenham, England

P. Ronan O'Connell, M.D., F.R.C.S.I.
Senior Registrar
Department of Surgery
Adelaide Hospital
Dublin, Ireland

**Humphrey J. O'Connor, M.D.,
 M.R.C.P.I.**
Consultant Physician
Department of Medicine
General Hospital
Tullamore, Ireland

Luke J. D. O'Donnell, M.D., M.R.C.P.I.
Senior Registrar, Honorary Lecturer
Department of Gastroenterology
St. Bartholomew's Hospital
London, England

**Colm A. O'Morain, M.D., M.Sc.,
 F.R.C.P.I.**
Consultant Gastroenterologist
Department of Gastroenterology
Meath/Adelaide Hospitals
Trinity College
Dublin, Ireland

A. S. Peña, M.D., Ph.D.
Associate Professor
Department of Gastroenterology
Leiden University Hospital
Leiden, The Netherlands

S. S. C. Rao, M.R.C.S., M.R.C.P., Ph.D.
Department of Gastroenterology
Royal Hallamshire Hospital
Sheffield, England

N. W. Read, M.D., F.R.C.P.
Professor
Centre for Human Nutrition
Northern General Hospital
Sheffield, England

**Peter J. Schoenberg, M.R.C.P., M.R.C.
 Psych.**
Department of Psychotherapy
Outpatient Department of Psychological
 Medicine
University College Hospital and
Consultant Psychotherapist and Honorary
 Senior Clinical Lecturer
Academic Department of Psychiatry
University College and Middlesex School
 of Medicine
London, England

S. Shivananda, Ph.D.
Department of Internal Medicine II
University Hospital Dijkreigt
Rotterdam, The Netherlands

Anne Tobin, M.R.C.P.I.
Research Fellow
Department of Gastroenterology
Meath/Adelaide Hospitals
Trinity College
Dublin, Ireland

**A. Brian West, M.B., M.S., M.R.C.
 Path.**
Assistant Professor and
Director of Gastrointestinal Pathology
Department of Pathology
Yale University School of Medicine
New Haven, Connecticut

To Marcelle, Cillian, Niall, and Cliodhna

TABLE OF CONTENTS

Chapter 1

EPIDEMIOLOGY OF ULCERATIVE COLITIS

A. S. Peña, S. Shivananda, and J. F. Mayberry

TABLE OF CONTENTS

I. INTRODUCTION

Epidemiological studies of inflammatory bowel diseases have been mainly concerned with the study of incidence and prevalence of the disease and demographic characteristics of the affected population. Most have been descriptive and only a few studies which have been analytical have addressed the question of etiology.

The reported incidence of ulcerative colitis in different populations varies with geographic area and period of study. Reported differences encountered in various studies may be due to the use of different methods of case ascertainment or, more interesting from the epidemiological point of view, they may reflect differences in lifestyle, diet, or other environmental factors. In reality, most studies are not directly comparable due to differences in period of study and methods of case ascertainment. The majority of reported studies have been retrospective and hospital based. Some of the differences in incidence may be explained by the exclusion of patients with only rectal involvement from a number of studies. Most early work was based on hospital admissions; however, more recent studies in well-defined communities have collected data on patients managed exclusively as outpatients or at home by their family practitioners.

Calkins and Mendeloff have extensively reviewed the different problems in epidemiologic approaches to inflammatory bowel disease.[1] Efforts to perform prospective- and community-based studies are justified for a disease with its highest incidence early in life, whose therapy may involve major surgery, and carries a high risk of developing intestinal cancer. Since ulcerative colitis may be due to a genetic predisposition triggered by environmental factors,[2] epidemiological studies designed to investigate such interactions may provide clues to its etiology.

II. INCIDENCE

The incidence of ulcerative colitis has now been reported from many different parts of the world (Table 1). Although ulcerative colitis is most common in northern Europe, the disease is now clearly seen with increasing frequency in southern Europe and also developing countries in other continents. The studies in Britain are inconsistent, with figures varying from $6.5/10^5$/year in Oxford to $15.1/10^5$/year in Tees.[3–5] This may reflect differences in case definition or methods of data collection. It could, however, be due to true regional variations or may even suggest a change in incidence over the last 20 years. In the Faroe islands and Norway the incidence has increased recently. These studies were prospective and included proctitis in the incidence calculation, both of which may have led to greater case ascertainment. Changes in incidence do occur. One of earliest such reports was that of Salem and Shubair[6] who described ulcerative colitis in Bedouin Arabs who had left their nomadic life in the desert and settled in the cities.

III. PREVALENCE

The majority of studies do not record true prevalence but only those symptomatic patients who contact the health care system over a 2- to 5-year period. The natural history of patients with proctitis only may be different from those with more extensive colitis cases and many may be omitted from studies of prevalence. In some patients the disease is only expressed for part of their life and the effect of this has not been fully evaluated.

The prevalence of ulcerative colitis and proctitis in areas of high risk, such as North Tees (England),[7] Copenhagen County,[8] and Iceland,[9] has been approximately 100 patients per 10^5 and as low as 6 patients per 10^5 in Bulgaria. In the Leiden region the prevalence was 58.4 per 10^5, which is similar to that in most other northern European countries.[10]

TABLE 1
Epidemiologic Studies of Ulcerative Colitis in Different Areas

Geographic area	Period of study	Incidence (10^5)
U.S.		
Minnesota	1935—1964	7.2
Baltimore, MD	1960—1963	4.6
Oxford, England	1951—1960	6.5
Cardiff, Wales	1968—1977	7.2
High Wycombe, England	1975—1984	7.1
North Tees, England	1971—1977	15.1
Aberdeen, Scotland	1967—1976	11.3
Denmark		
Copenhagen County	1962—1978	8.1
Copenhagen County	1981—1988	9.5
Faroe Islands	1964—1983	7.5
Faroe Islands[a]	1981—1988	20.3
Iceland	1950—1959	2.8
Iceland	1970—1979	7.4
Norway	1946—1969	2.4
Bergen (western Norway)	1976—1980	10.0
Western Norway[a]	1984—1985	14.8
Leiden, The Netherlands	1979—1983	6.8
Sweden		
Stockholm County	1975—1979	4.3
West Germany		
Marburg-Lahn	1962—1975	5.1
Ruhr	1980—1984	2.9
Tel Aviv, Israel	1961—1970	3.6
Borsod, Hungary	1972—1983	3.1

[a] Prospective studies.

IV. DEMOGRAPHIC CHARACTERISTICS

A. AGE
In most studies ulcerative colitis has shown a bimodal age distribution in the white population.

B. SEX
There is no predominance of the disease in either sex.

C. RACE
Several studies have shown that Jews have a higher incidence than the other races living in the same area. This was first shown in Baltimore in 1960 to 1963[11] where Jews had an annual incidence of 13 per 10^5 compared with non-Jewish whites (3.8 per 10^5) and blacks (1.4 per 10^5). Similar figures have been observed in the Cape Town area of South Africa where Jews had an incidence of 17, Whites of 5, coloreds of 1.4, and blacks of 0.6 per 10^5 (Table 2).[12]

D. MIGRANTS
In the new Negev in southern Israel, 58% of the population are immigrants. It has recently been reported that Jews of European and American origin have a significantly higher incidence (10.8 per 10^5) than those Jews born in North Africa and the Middle East (5.1 per 10^5) or in Israel (4.1 per 10^5).[13] This study suggests that environmental influences play an important

TABLE 2
Epidemiologic Studies of Ulcerative Colitis in
Different Ethnic Groups

	Period of study	Incidence (cases/10^5 population/year)	Ref.
South Africa	1980—1984		12
Jews		17.0	
Whites		5.0	
Colored		1.9	
Blacks		0.6	

TABLE 3
Incidence of Ulcerative Colitis by Urban and
Agrarian Municipalities in the Area of
Leiden, The Netherlands (1979—1983)

Municipal groups	Population at risk	Population density per km²	Incidence per 10^5
A	76,866 (17%)[a]	551	8.8
B	206,253 (47%)[a]	1,165	4.8
C	156,682 (36%)[a]	2,820	8.6

[a] % of total population.

role in the development of ulcerative colitis. In the Netherlands, there has been a significant migration of people of Indonesian, Turkish, Moroccan, and Surinamese origin into areas such as Leiden.[10] The migration is recent (25 to 30 years) and the epidemiology of chronic disease in these groups is not yet clear. A study in Leiden identified six cases of proctocolitis among the 7037 migrants, compared with none of Crohn's disease. The prevalence of ulcerative colitis in migrants was 85.3 per 10^5 (range = 35 to 195, 95% confidence limits) and this was not significantly different from the indigenous Dutch population.[10]

E. URBAN-RURAL DISTRIBUTION

Although urban and rural differences in the incidence and prevalence of ulcerative colitis have been reported, the categories of urban and rural have not been clearly defined. In the Netherlands all municipal areas are classified into A, agrarian municipalities, B, bedroom suburbs, and C, cities, by the Central Bureau of Statistics.[14] This classification is based on the (1) characteristics of the settlement as reflected in the density of housing and population, (2) the characteristics of the occupation of a significant proportion of its labor force, and (3) the social and economic functions of the settlement. Table 3 shows the difference in incidence in such urban and rural areas in the Leiden Health Care Region in the Netherlands. People living in dormitory suburbs were at significantly less risk than those in towns or the country but this cannot be attributed to differences in population density. Environmental factors, such as different water supplies, fail to explain these differences; however, there may be a role for other environmental factors in the etiology of ulcerative colitis. In northern Alberta, Canada it has been found that there is no urban vs. rural effect for ulcerative colitis, whereas a striking effect was seen in Crohn's disease, and in these areas the prevalence of Crohn's disease was higher than that for ulcerative colitis.[15]

F. SOCIOECONOMIC FACTORS

Bonnevie found that Danish patients with ulcerative colitis were more often from the senior-salaried section of society than would be expected.[16] Similar observations have been made in the U.S.[17]

V. FAMILIAL AGGREGATIONS

It has long been known that the familial occurrence of ulcerative colitis and Crohn's disease is increased in patients with ulcerative colitis. A general prevalence of 7.9% of familial occurrences was found in an unselected population in a well-defined area over a long period of time (Stockholm county, Sweden).[18] Recently, age-corrected empiric risk estimates for inflammatory bowel disease in the Ashkenazi Jewish population in the U.S. has been developed.[19] This study demonstrates that there is an increased risk of ulcerative colitis for the offspring, siblings, and parents who have a positive family history. Of patients with ulcerative colitis, 19.8% had a positive family history. In the study of the Stockholm county,[18] patients with a positive family history of ulcerative colitis were also found to have a lower age at onset of the disease; this was not the case in the study from Los Angeles, CA.[19]

A. FIRST-DEGREE RELATIVES

The prevalence of ulcerative colitis in first-degree relatives was found to be 15 times higher than in nonrelatives and the prevalence of Crohn's disease in these patients was 3.5 times higher than in nonrelatives.[18]

B. TWINS

In another recent study from Sweden,[20] based on retrieval of all twins and all patients with the diagnosis of inflammatory bowel disease in the population, it was found that in ulcerative colitis only one of 16 monozygotic twin pairs was concordant for the disease, that is 6.3%, significantly lower than the rate of concordance found for Crohn's disease, which was 8 out of 18 (44.4%). This finding suggests that evaluations based on earlier reports of twins with ulcerative colitis where a higher degree of concordance had been observed probably overestimated the importance of genetic factors in this disease.

C. SPOUSES

Very few cases of ulcerative colitis in husband and wife have been reported. In some of the couples, one of the couple was affected with Crohn's disease instead of ulcerative colitis.[21,22] If the shared familial environment factors were sufficient for the expression of the disease, many more cases should exist.

D. SUMMARY

In summary, the studies performed in families of patients with ulcerative colitis indicated that genetic factors play a role in the etiology of ulcerative colitis. Genetic factors seem to be necessary but are not sufficient to develop the disease.

VI. ENVIRONMENTAL FACTORS

A. DIETARY FACTORS

High meat and fat consumption have been reported as factors. Interestingly, in the Faroe Islands high fat consumption has significantly increased in recent years. As was shown above, these islands have the highest incidence of ulcerative colitis in the world (Table 1). The roles of dietary practices, water supply, agrarian and urban areas, smoking habits, and other social activities are yet to be clearly defined.[23]

B. SMOKING

There are many studies showing that the relative risk of ulcerative colitis developing in nonsmokers is definitely higher compared with smokers.[24,25] Ex-smokers usually develop their disease after stopping smoking.[26,27] Epidemiological studies consistently support the different association of cigarette smoking with ulcerative colitis and Crohn's disease. It has been suggested that in genetically predisposed individuals, the smoking exposure may determine the type of inflammatory bowel disease that will develop.[27] The study of identical twins in Sweden showed that the smoking pattern was similar in concordant and discordant twins. After the time of diagnosis, two healthy monozygotic twins had given up smoking for a mean period of 6.5 years without developing ulcerative colitis. This implies that the sharing of identical genes and smoking patterns is not enough.[20] Other environmental factors should be investigated.

C. CONTRACEPTIVE PILL

Oral contraceptive users have a definite increased risk for Crohn's disease but not for ulcerative colitis.[28]

D. SUMMARY

In summary, the environmental factors so far identified, such as dietary factors, smoking patterns, and the use of oral contraceptive pills appear to be more important as risk factors for developing Crohn's disease than for ulcerative colitis. In a recent international case control study, 197 patients with ulcerative colitis, whose disease started before the age of 20 years and whose age at time of study was less than 25 years, were compared with two age- and sex-matched controls for each patient. No significant differences were found between patients and controls in relation to various human and nonhuman contacts during childhood. Number of siblings, being an only child, and birth order did not differ between patients and controls.[29]

VII. RISK OF CANCER

The cumulative cancer risk rates of ulcerative colitis in population studies have been found to be lower than those reported from major medical centers. One of the most recent studies performed in the central area of Israel has shown a 0.2% cumulative incidence of colorectal cancer at 10 years and 5.5% at 20 years.[30]

VIII. MORTALITY

The mortality of the disease is low. This has been particularly evident in those studies comprehending a properly defined community.

A recent study from England has shown that mortality from ulcerative colitis in district hospitals is low in patients who are regularly followed; however, there is a risk of late colonic carcinomas in those now reviewed in the clinic.[5] This study has suggested that colonoscopic surveillance is necessary and feasible.

IX. FUTURE STUDIES

Since most of the observed geographic variation may be due to data collection occurring at different times in different places during years when the disease may be changing, in the future, definition of epidemiologically operational criteria of ulcerative colitis should be used as an essential part of the standardized research methodology in simultaneous prospective studies, developing methods to ensure complete ascertainment of incident cases of ulcerative colitis within the areas of study. A recent study from Nottingham[31] has suggested that studies which are based on symptomatic patients diagnosed in the hospital may underestimate the true prevalence of ulcerative colitis by approximately 30%. These authors were able to identify previously undiagnosed asymptomatic cases of inflammatory bowel disease as a result of a population screening study for the detection of colorectal neoplasia using a fecal occult blood test. None of these patients had sought medical advice because of abdominal pain, diarrhea, or rectal bleeding. These findings are relevant for the epidemiology of ulcerative colitis and Crohn's disease, and efforts should be made toward the identification of such patients. Cohort studies in well-defined regions, especially in areas of migration of large groups, such as in Israel, may give evidence supporting the presence of environmental factors in the etiology of the disease and, hopefully, clues to identify environmental factors other than those already discussed.

REFERENCES

1. **Calkins, B.M. and Mendeloff, Al.,** Epidemiology of inflammatory bowel disease, *Epidem. Rev.,* 8, 60, 1986.
2. **Kirsner, J.B.,** Inflammatory bowel disease. Considerations of etiology and pathogenesis, *Am. J. Gastroenterol.,* 69, 253, 1978.
3. **Evans, J.G. and Acheson, E.D.,** An epidemiological study of ulcerative colitis and regional enteritis in the Oxford area, *Gut,* 6, 311, 1965.
4. **Morris, T.J. and Rhodes, J.,** Incidence of proctocolitis in the Cardiff region 1968-77, *Gut,* 21, A923, 1980.
5. **Jones, H.W., Grogono, J., and Hoare, A.M.,** Surveillance in ulcerative colitis: burdens and benefit, *Gut,* 29, 325, 1988.
6. **Salem, S.N. and Shubair, K.S.,** Non-specific ulcerative colitis in Bedouin Arabs, *Lancet,* i, 473, 1967.
7. **Devlin, H.B., Datta, D., and Dellipiani, A.W.,** The incidence and prevalence of inflammatory bowel disease in North Tees health district, *World J. Surg.,* 4, 183, 1980.
8. **Binder, V., Both, H., Hansen, P.K., Hendriksen, C., Kreiner, S., and Torp-Pendersen, K.,** Incidence and prevalence of ulcerative colitis and Crohn's disease in the County of Copenhagen 1962—1978, *Gastroenterology,* 83, 563, 1982.
9. **Skarstein, A., Arnesjo, B., Burhol, P., Nordgard, K., Borkje, B., Fluge, G., and Haug, K.,** *Scand. J. Gastroenterol.,* 17 (Abstr.) (Suppl. 18), 349, 1982.
10. **Shivananda, S., Peña, A.S., Mayberry, J.F., Ruitenberg, E.J., and Hoedemaeker, Ph.J.,** Epidemiology of proctocolitis in the region of Leiden, The Netherlands, *Scand. J. Gastroenterol.,* 22, 993, 1988.
11. **Monk, M., Mendeloff, Al., Siegel, C.I., and Lilienfeld, A.,** An epidemiological study of ulcerative colitis and regional enteritis among adults in Baltimore. I. Hospital incidence and prevalence, 1960—1963, *Gastroenterology,* 53, 198, 1967.
12. **Wright, J.P., Frogatti, J., O'Keffe, E.A., Ackerman, S., Watermeyer, S., Louw, J., Adams, G., Girwood, A.H., Burns, D.G., and Marks, I.N.,** The epidemiology of inflammatory bowel disease in Cape Town 1980—1984, *S. Afr. Med. J.,* 70, 10, 1986.
13. **Odes, H.S., Fraser, D., and Kraiec, J.,** Inflammatory bowel disease in migrant and native Jewish populations of southern Israel, *Dig. Dis. Sci.,* 31 (Suppl. 835 nr), 322, 1986.
14. Central Bureau of Statistics (CBS), Typologie van de Nederlandse gemeenten naar urbanisatiegraad, Staatsuitgeverij, The Hague 1979—1983.
15. **Pinchbeck, B.R., Kirdeikis, J., and Thomson, A.B.R.,** Inflammatory bowel disease in northern Alberta, *J. Clin. Gastroenterol.,* 10, 505, 1988.
16. **Bonnevie, O.,** A socio-economic study of patients with ulcerative colitis, *Scand. J. Gastroenterol.,* 2, 129, 1967.
17. **Monk, M., Mendeloff, A.I., Siegel, C.I., and Lilienfeld, A.,** An epidemiological study of ulcerative colitis and regional enteritis among adults in Baltimore. II. Social and demographic factors, *Gastroenterology,* 56, 847, 1969.
18. **Monsén, U., Broström, O., Nordenvall, B., Sörstad, J., and Hellers, G.,** Prevalence of inflammatory bowel disease among relatives of patients with ulcerative colitis, *Scand. J. Gastroenterol.,* 22, 214, 1987.
19. **Roth, M.P., Petersen, G.M., McElree, C., Vadheim, C.M., Panish, J.F., and Rotter, J.I.,** Familial empiric risk estimates of inflammatory bowel disease in Ashkenazi Jews, *Gastroenterology,* 96, 1016, 1989.

20. **Tysk, C., Lindberg, E., Järnerot, G., and Flodérus-Myrhed, B.,** Ulcerative colitis and Crohn's disease in an unselected population of monozygotic and dizygotic twins. A study of heritability and the influence of smoking, *Gut,* 29, 990, 1988.

21. **Craxi, A., Oliva, L., and Di Stefano, G.,** Ulcerative colitis in a married couple, *Ital. J. Gastroenterol.,* 11, 184, 1979.

22. **Almy, T.P. and Sherlock, P.,** Genetic aspects of ulcerative colitis and regional enteritis, *Gastroenterology,* 51, 757, 1966.

23. **Penny, W.J., Penny, E., Mayberry, J.F., and Rhodes, J.,** Mormons, smoking and ulcerative colitis, *Lancet,* ii, 1315, 1983.

24. **Smith, M.B., Lashner, B.A., and Hanauer, S.B.,** Smoking and inflammatory bowel disease in families, *Am. J. Gastroenterol.,* 83, 407, 1988.

25. **Katschinski, B., Logan, R.F.A., Edmond, M., and Langman, M.J.S.,** Smoking and sugar intake are separate but interactive risk factors in Crohn's disease, *Gut,* 29, 1202, 1988.

26. **Boyko, E.J., Perera, D.R., Koepsell, T.D., Keane, E.M., and Inui, T.S.,** Effects of cigarette smoking on the clinical course of ulcerative colitis, *Scand. J. Gastroenterol.,* 23, 1147, 1988.

27. **Tobin, M.V., Logan, R.F.A., Langman, M.J.S., McConnell, R.B., and Gilmore, I.T.,** Cigarette smoking and inflammatory bowel disease, *Gastroenterology,* 93, 316, 1987.

28. **Calkins, B.M., Mendeloff, A.I., and Garland, C.,** Inflammatory bowel disease in oral contraceptive users (letter), *Gastroenterology,* 91, 523, 1986.

29. **Gilat, T., Hacohen, D., Lilos, P., and Langman, M.J.S.,** Childhood factors in ulcerative colitis and Crohn's disease, An international cooperative study, *Scand. J. Gastroenterol.,* 22, 1009, 1987.

30. **Gilat, T., Fireman, Z., Grossman, A., Hacohen, D., Kadish, U., Ron, E., Rozen, P., and Lilos, P.,** Colorectal cancer in patients with ulcerative colitis. A population study in central Israel, *Gastroenterology,* 94, 870, 1988.

31. **Mayberry, J.F., Ballantyne, K.C., Hardcastle, J.D., Mangham, C., and Pye, G.,** Epidemiological study of asymptomatic inflammatory bowel disease: the identification of cases during a screening programme for colorectal cancer, *Gut,* 30, 481, 1989.

32. **Róin, F. and Róin, J.,** Inflammatory bowel disease of the Faroe Islands, 1981-1988. A prospective epidemiological study: primary report, *Scand. J. Gastroenterol.,* 24(Suppl. 170), 44, 1989.

32. **Björnsson, S.,** Inflammatory bowel disease in Iceland during a 30-year period, 1950-1979, *Scand. J. Gastroenterol.,* 24(Suppl. 170), 47, 1989.

34. **Hang, K., Schrumpf, E., Barstad, S., Fluge, G., Halvorsen, J. F., and The study group of inflammatory bowel disease in Western Norway,** Epidemiology of ulcerative colitis in Western Norway, *Scand. J. Gastroenterol.,* 23, 517, 1988.

Chapter 2

ADHESIVE *E. COLI* IN ULCERATIVE COLITIS

D. A. Burke and A. T. R. Axon

TABLE OF CONTENTS

I. INTRODUCTION

The view that bacteria may play a role in the pathogenesis of ulcerative colitis was suggested by Sir Arthur Hurst[1] and is supported by a number of clinical observations and animal experiments. The clinical features of ulcerative colitis in relapse closely resemble those of infectious colitis which may be caused by a variety of enteric pathogens. Moreover, the disease is limited to the mucosa of the colon which is most intimately associated with an abundant microbial flora. Experimentally, it has proved difficult to induce colitis in germ-free animals[1] and prophylactic treatment with antibiotics in these studies prevents its development.[2,3] Consequently, over the years a great deal of research has been undertaken in an attempt to identify a microbial cause for ulcerative colitis in man.

II. *ESCHERICHIA COLI*

A number of microorganisms have been proposed as potential pathogens in ulcerative colitis (Table 1); however, supportive evidence is lacking in the majority. Interest in *Escherichia coli* as a possible etiological factor has arisen not only because it is the predominant aerobic bacterium in the adult fecal flora, but because it is also a well-recognized primary intestinal pathogen.[4]

Quantitative comparisons of fecal coliforms in ulcerative colitis and control groups have produced conflicting data.[5,8] There are several methodological reasons why this may have occurred, including differences in sampling and culture techniques and the fact that diarrhea from any cause may alter the proportions of viable bacteria isolated.[9] A different and possibly more relevant approach is to study qualitative differences between the organism found in the feces of patients with ulcerative colitis and controls.

III. QUALITATIVE DIFFERENCES OF FECAL *E. COLI* IN ULCERATIVE COLITIS

Cooke, in 1968, demonstrated that fecal *E. coli* from patients with ulcerative colitis differed from control isolates in that they were more likely to produce hemolysin and necrotoxin and more commonly possessed the ability to dilate rabbit ileal loops.[10] Subsequent studies, however, suggested that the appearance of strains with the ability to produce hemolysin and necrotoxin tended to follow the onset of relapse, suggesting that they might have been acquired as a result of the disease process.[11]

Further indirect evidence in favor of *E. coli* having a role in ulcerative colitis comes from the immunological abnormalities that can be found in this disorder. Higher titers of antibodies to *E. coli* O antigens are present in patients with ulcerative colitis compared with controls,[12] and antibodies to *E. coli* 014, which are found more commonly in patients with ulcerative colitis, cross-react with colonic epithelium.[13] More significantly, cellular cytotoxicity to colonic epithelium can be induced in lymphocytes exposed to an *E. coli* lipopolysaccharide extract.[14]

IV. THE ADHESIVE PROPERTY OF PATHOGENIC *E. COLI*

Although five distinct groups of diarrheagenic *E. coli* are now recognized[4] (Table 2), a number of studies have emphasized the importance of mucosal adhesion as a virulence factor in these organisms both in animals and man.[15-17] Satterwhite and colleagues, in their studies of enterotoxigenic *E. coli* (ETEC), demonstrated in man that toxin production alone was insufficient to produce disease in all cases.[16] Using a laboratory-derived strain that retained the ability to produce toxin but lacked the mucosal adhesive property they confirmed by oral challenge that the parent strain caused diarrhea but that the laboratory derivative did not.

TABLE 1
Microbial Agents Proposed and
Investigated as Etiological Agents
in Ulcerative Colitis

Recognized pathogens
  Escherichia coli
  Shigella spp.
  Salmonella spp.
  Clostridium difficile
  Entamoeba histolytica
  Chlamydia spp.
  Cryptosporidia
  Campylobacter spp.
   Viruses
Others
  Bacteroides spp. (*Bacteroides necrophorus*)
  Streptococcus spp.
  Geotrichum spp.

Colonization by ETEC is dependent upon mucosal adhesion which is mediated by pilus-like filamentous protein structures that bind to specific receptors on the cell membrane. Several antigenically distinct and species-specific fimbrial antigens have been identified.[18] Nonpathogenic strains of *E. coli* may possess pilus-like appendages (type I pili). However, the fimbrial antigens of enterotoxigenic *E. coli* can be differentiated from type I pili by their ability to hemagglutinate the red blood cells of different animal species and adhere *in vitro* to a variety of cell substrates in the presence of the sugar D-mannose.[19] This mannose-resistant hemagglutination (MRHA) of different species of red blood cells can differentiate between the colonization factors I and II of human ETEC.[20]

The genetic determinants controlling the production of these *E. coli*-adhesive factors are carried on extrachromasomal DNA in the form of plasmids which may be transferable to other strains.[17,21,22] Although the pathogenic strains appear to be restricted to a limited number of serotypes, the virulence of the organism is often dependant on the presence of DNA that may be transferred between cells; consequently, serotyping alone is insufficient to indicate the pathogenicity of a strain.

The mechanisms whereby nontoxin-producing enteropathogenic *E. coli* (EPEC) cause diarrhea is not fully understood; however, in these, too, mannose-resistant adhesion appears to be an essential factor in the mediation of their pathogenicity.[4,17] The importance of adhesion as a virulence factor for *E. coli* is also recognized in nongastrointestinal disease, such as the urinary tract.[23] Indeed, the intimate mucosal association of bacterium and cell surface appears to be a prerequisite for colonization and initiation of disease in a wide range of intestinal pathogens including the other groups of diarrheagenic *E. coli*.[4]

Although the possession of an adhesive property does not in itself confer a pathogenic role, it does appear to be an important prerequisite for pathogenic *E. coli,* so the finding of *E. coli* with adhesive properties in the feces of patients with ulcerative colitis could be of etiological and therapeutic importance.

V. *E. COLI* WITH ADHESIVE PROPERTIES IN ULCERATIVE COLITIS

Dickinson et al., in 1980, were the first to report an increased prevalence of fecal coliforms with *in vitro* adhesive and invasive properties in patients with ulcerative colitis.[24] They examined the ability of *E. coli* to adhere to or invade HeLa cells in tissue culture and found that 35% of patients with active ulcerative colitis and 27% of those in remission were

TABLE 2
The Distinct Categories of
***E. coli* that Produce Diarrhea**

1. Enterotoxigenic	(ETEC)
2. Enteropathogenic	(EPEC)
3. Enteroinvasive	(ETEC)
4. Enterohaemorrhagic	(EHEC)
5. Enteroadherent	(EAEC)

colonized by adhesive or invasive fecal coliform, compared to only 5% of a control group. One serotype tended to predominate in patients with ulcerative colitis; this was usually an adhesive or invasive strain, whereas a greater variety of strains was encountered in the controls. Only two of the adhesive/invasive strains in the patients with ulcerative colitis were of a recognized pathogenic serotype; however, the limitations of ascribing pathogenicity by serotyping alone have been alluded to already.

It would be premature to ascribe a primary pathogenic role to those organisms simply on the basis of *in vitro* qualitative differences. The presence of adhesive *E. coli* in the stool of patients with ulcerative colitis could be an incidental finding, and they may not have a direct pathogenic role; the inflammatory process within the colon may result in the exposure of receptors that would otherwise be masked. This mechanism could then result in the selection of strains with an appropriate adhesin. Evidence for this type of response comes from the demonstration of enhanced adhesion to red blood cells by *Actinomyces viscosus* and *A. naeslundii* following treatment of the red cells with the enzyme neuraminidase.[26] This treatment removes sialic acid exposing the appropriate receptors. A similar response has been shown by *E. coli* in urinary tract infection where treatment of the bladder mucosa with neuraminidase increased their adhesion.[26] This same "unmasking" effect could operate for *E. coli* in the colon of colitics secondary to the action of host or bacterial enzymes.

Further research has been performed to extend these initial findings in ulcerative colitis and to explore whether these organisms are primary or secondary.

Using the HeLa cell assay, Pinder et al. examined *E. coli* isolated from patients presenting in their first attack of ulcerative colitis and compared them with those obtained from others during relapse of established disease.[27] They found a greater proportion of adhesive strains in those with a first attack. If damage to the intestinal mucosa was the prime reason for the presence of these organisms it might be expected that the patients with chronic and often long-standing disease would have shown an increased incidence of adhesive strains.

Recognized adhesins of *E. coli* are not only species specific but they demonstrate somatotropic localization because of the presence of specific receptors on the cell surface of the target organ.[28,29] Therefore, the HeLa cell assay using neoplastic cells originally obtained from the genital tract has several disadvantages in the investigation of intestinal adherence, especially as enzymatic stripping methods are used in the manipulation of the cell line. These factors could result in the expression of nonphysiological receptors for bacteria.

Dickinson et al. attempted to demonstrate adhesion of colitic *E. coli* isolates to the target organ of ulcerative colitis by incubating them with explant cultures of rectal tissue from patients with ulcerative colitis and controls.[30] They were unable to demonstrate adhesion to rectal mucosa, even when using recognized pathogenic strains known to adhere *in vivo*. This could have been a methodological problem with the explant rectal culture assay, possibly due to the profuse mucus production that occurs with these cultures. We have made further attempts along similar lines to demonstrate adhesion of colitic *E. coli* using colonoscopic biopsies and a greater number of *E. coli* isolates (unpublished observations), but again with negative results.

VI. USE OF A BUCCAL EPITHELIAL CELL PREPARATION

In an attempt to confirm the observations of Dickinson et al. using a cell substrate with a closer association to the intestinal tract than HeLa cells, we have studied *E. coli* adhesion using buccal epithelial cells.[31] This method has several advantages. It is a quantitative method and, as buccal epithelial cells can easily be obtained from patients, it allows the assessment of host factors that may influence bacterial adhesion. Buccal epithelial cells do appear to express receptors similar to those of the intestine, as ETEC can be cultured from the oropharynx of children who are infected with these pathogens.[32] Finally, an adhesive *E. coli* has been shown to have a similar degree of adhesion for buccal epithelial cells and fetal enterocytes.[33] These data suggest that this technique may be particularly suitable for the study of fecal *E. coli* thought to have adhesive properties.

To date there is no evidence to suggest that type I pilus adhesion is associated with intestinal pathogenicity in man. In the HeLa cell adhesion assay studies reported previously, adhesion mediated by type I pilus was not excluded. Therefore, in the buccal epithelial cell adhesion assay, D-mannose was included in the preparation during incubation in order to eliminate this factor. In addition, the bacterial strains tested were grown on solid media because type I pili are best developed when grown in liquid media.

After incubation of buccal epithelial cells with a suspension of test bacterium, nonadherent bacteria are removed by washing over a 5-μm filter. An impression smear of the buccal cells was then dried, fixed, and stained by Gram's method. The degree of mannose-resistant adhesion is determined by inspecting 100 nonoverlapping cells in at least 10 high-power fields and determining the proportion of cells with more than 50 adherent Gram-negative rods (Figure 1). An adhesion index (percent buccal epithelial cell) is derived by subtracting the count obtained from a control culture without added bacteria.

Results using the buccal epithelial cell technique confirm that patients with ulcerative colitis do harbor *E. coli* with a mannose-resistant adhesive property, the adhesion indices of the colitic *E. coli* (median 43.5%) being significantly higher than those from controls (2%), $p < 0.0001$ (Figure 2).

In these initial studies, all colitic isolates were more adhesive than any control isolate, suggesting that the true incidence of adhesive *E. coli* in this disease is higher than the 35% reported by Dickinson et al. using HeLa cells.[24] When buccal epithelial cells from differing sources were studied, *E. coli* isolates from colitic patients were shown to have no greater affinity for the cells derived from their host or for those of other colitic patients and controls (Figures 3 and 4).

When the buccal epithelial and HeLa cell adhesion assays were compared, the results confirmed that the buccal epithelial cell technique is more sensitive in detecting adhesive *E. coli* in ulcerative colitis;[34] however, both methods showed a significant difference between colitic and control *E. coli* isolates based on their adhesive property. All HeLa cell-positive strains (Figure 5) were buccal epithelial cell adhesion positive (i.e., adhesion index >25%); however, the HeLa cell method failed to identify 32% of buccal epithelial cell adhesion-positive strains. If both methods measure the same adhesive property then the HeLa cell method is considerably less sensitive. In all buccal epithelial cell adhesion assays performed control standard, nonadhesive *E. coli* strains, together with all wild strains obtained from control subjects, had adhesion indices of <25%. This indicates that the increased numbers of adhesion-positive strains detected in the colitic patients was not due to a loss of specificity. When *E. coli* isolates from a larger number of colitics (n = 59) were examined, it was found that not all colitic isolates demonstrated buccal epithelial cell adhesion. However adhesive strains were found in colitics in remission and in patients with Crohn's disease.[35] In fact, 86% of *E. coli* isolates from patients with inflammatory bowel disease were adhesion positive compared with none of the controls (Figure 6).

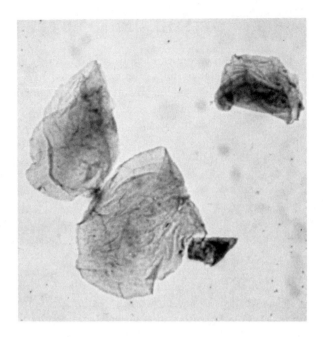

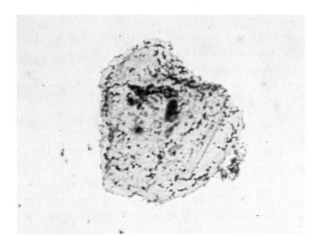

FIGURE 1. Adhesive *E. coli* from a patient with ulcerative colitis attached to buccal epithelial cells.

VII. ADHESIVE *E. COLI* IN OTHER INFLAMMATORY COLITIDES

Controversy exists as to whether Crohn's disease and ulcerative colitis are separate disease entities or different ends of the spectrum of the same disease. It is therefore very interesting that adhesive *E. coli* were found in both conditions in similar proportions. Of course, it may be that the mucosal inflammation which exists in both conditions predisposes both groups to colonization with these organisms. On the other hand, in the same study, *E. coli* isolated from patients with infections recognized as causing colonic inflammation were also studied. The median buccal epithelial cell adhesion index for *E. coli* from those with infectious diarrhea was only 14% as compared to 43% for *E. coli* from patients with a relapse of ulcerative colitis

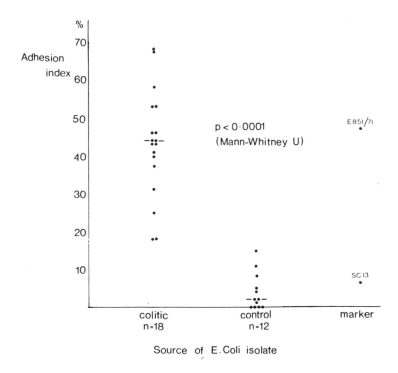

FIGURE 2. The buccal epithelial cell adhesion indices of *E. coli* isolated from patients with ulcerative colitis and controls (single source of buccal epithelial cells).

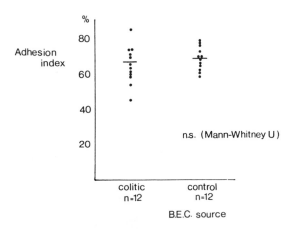

FIGURE 3. Adhesion of an adhesive *E. coli* strain to buccal epithelial cells obtained from colitic patients and controls.

($p < 0.005$). Only 27% of *E. coli* from the infectious diarrhea group were adhesion positive as defined by an adhesion index >25% compared with 86% in the inflammatory bowel disease group. This carriage rate is nevertheless greater than one would expect in a normal control population. Dickinson et al. found that only 5% of patients with other types of colitis, including pseudomembranous colitis, were carrying an adhesive strain, a similar incidence to that of controls in the HeLa cell study.[24]

Could the presence of these adhesive organisms be due to previous treatment of ulcerative

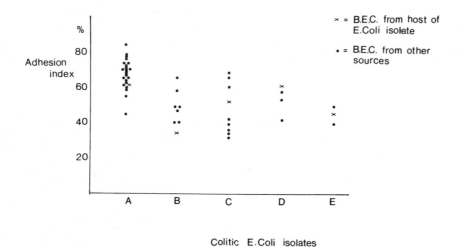

FIGURE 4.   Adhesion of *E. coli* isolated from patients with ulcerative colitis to their host buccal epithelial cells and those from other sources.

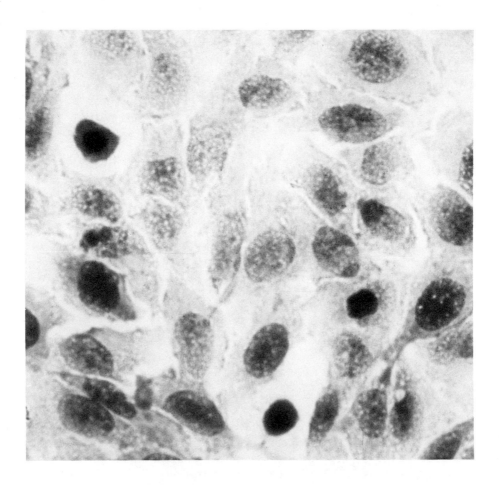

FIGURE 5a.   Adhesion of *E. coli* to HeLa cells.

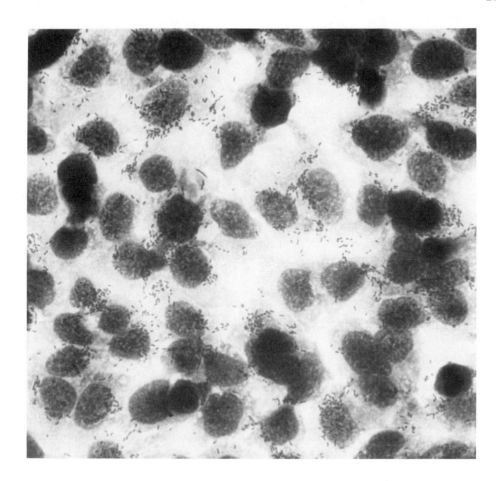

FIGURE 5b. Adhesion of *E. coli* to HeLa cells.

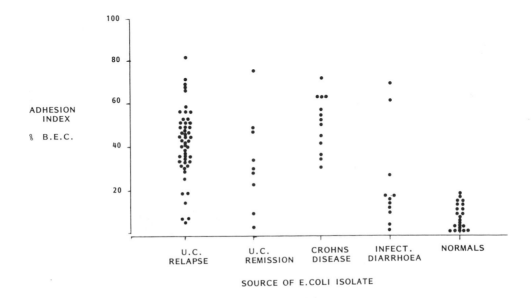

FIGURE 6. Buccal epithelial cell adhesion indices of *E. coli* obtained from various sources.

colitis? Sulfasalazine has an antibiotic component which might result in the selection of resistant strains of bacteria[36] that may also possess an adhesive property.

This appears unlikely; *E. coli* with adhesive properties are found in patients presenting in their first attack and this includes some who have received no treatment. Furthermore, the association of colitis and adhesive *E. coli* is unaffected by a history of current or past administration of sulfasalazine or sulfonamide resistance in the fecal *E. coli* of colitics.[27,35,37]

The nature of the adhesin possessed by *E. coli* isolated in ulcerative colitis is unknown. Bacteria-to-cell interactions are complex and varied, but include lectin-like, electrostatic, and hydrophobic mechanisms. When the surface hydrophobicity of a bacterial cell is reduced the cell surface charge is reduced, diminishing the repulsive forces that exist between negatively charged bodies, increasing the chance that adhesion may occur.[38] Bacterial adhesins can be ranked on the basis of their surface hydrophobicity with recognized adhesive and pathogenic *E. coli,* showing a greater surface hydrophobicity than nonpathogens.[39]

The hydrophobic properties of *E. coli* from patients with ulcerative colitis have been assessed by the salting-out method of Lindahl et al.[39] and compared with that of *E. coli* from controls.[40] Using this method, colitic *E. coli* were found to be significantly more hydrophobic than control *E. coli*. The salting-out score correlated negatively with the buccal epithelial cell adhesion index, and when *E. coli* were grown at 18°C both properties were temporarily reduced suggesting that the two properties are related to each other. The salting-out method again clearly differentiated the majority of colitic *E. coli* isolates from those of controls. Mannose-resistant adhesion in pathogenic *E. coli* is mediated by both fimbrial and afimbrial mechanisms; however, in either case, there is an increase in surface hydrophobicity.[41] Ljungh and Wadstrom[42] reported that 31% of their colitic *E. coli* isolates expressed surface hydrophobicity. In this study they also reported subepithelial connective tissue protein binding of *E. coli* isolated from patients with ulcerative colitis. This adhesive property was demonstrated by the agglutination of latex particles coated with fibronectin, collagen type II, or fibrinogen. However, this connective tissue adhesive property did not correlate with surface hydrophobicity and was detectable in strains grown at 20°C, suggesting that this property is probably distinct from the HeLa and buccal epithelial cell adhesive property which is lost when strains are grown at 18°C.[40] They suggest however that these strains are likely to have a selective advantage enabling them to colonize colonic lesions and maybe retard the healing process.

Hemagglutination studies of *E. coli* isolated from ulcerative colitis patients have not as yet identified any recognized mannose-resistant fimbrial adhesions;[42,44] however, 42% of isolates express a mannose-resistant hemagglutinin.[44] Type I pili were found less commonly among isolates from patients with ulcerative colitis than controls in one study; however, the significance of this finding is unknown.[43] Indeed, the colonization factor antigens, CFAI and CFAII, identifiable by hemagglutination, demonstrate somatotropic localization resulting in colonization of the small bowel and might not necessarily be involved in the pathogenesis of colonic disease.

VIII. DOES ERADICATION OF *E. COLI* IN ULCERATIVE COLITIS IMPROVE OUTCOME?

The qualitative differences in *E. coli* from patients with ulcerative colitis compared with controls, which have been identified by ourselves and others, raises the possibility that they might be involved in the pathogenesis of the disease. It is neither practical nor ethical (at least in man) to fullfil all of Koch's postulates for these organisms in ulcerative colitis. However, if their eradication were to result in clinical improvement it would support the hypothesis.

Complete and permanent eradication of gut organisms is almost impossible to achieve safely. However, we have recently assessed the benefit of temporary eradication of *E. coli* from patients with ulcerative colitis using oral tobramycin as an adjunct to standard therapy.

In a preliminary study, 7-d absorption of orally administered tobramycin was shown to be no greater from inflamed bowel than normal bowel.[45]

A double-blind placebo-controlled trial was undertaken comparing adjunctive oral tobramycin given for 7 d with placebo. A total of 84 patients with acute colitis were recruited. All of the original strains of *E. coli* were eradicated from 82% of the tobramycin-treated group compared with only 9% of the placebo group.[46] At the endpoint of the trial, 74% of those patients who had received tobramycin were completely asymptomatic compared with only 43% of the placebo group ($p < 0.008$). This clinical response was mirrored by a significant histological improvement ($p < 0.05$).

Ten patients in each group presented in their first attack, all of those receiving tobramycin, achieved complete symptomatic remission during the trial period compared with only six in the placebo group. No side effects were encountered with oral tobramycin and bacterial resistance to tobramycin did not emerge in those treated with this aminoglycoside.

A few controlled trials of antibiotic therapy in ulcerative colitis have been reported but this is the first to demonstrate any benefit. It would be wrong to conclude that the better results obtained in the tobramycin group are necessarily the result of eliminating *E. coli* with adhesive properties; other factors may have been responsible. Nevertheless, the findings are consistent with the theory that *E. coli* may play a role in ulcerative colitis. Other possibilities are that it may cause a reduction in chemotactic peptides[44] or perhaps some effect unrelated to its antimicrobial activity.

IX. SUMMARY

In vitro studies demonstrating qualitative differences between the *E. coli* isolated from patients with ulcerative colitis and controls, together with the therapeutic response to oral tobramycin, raise the possibility that these organisms play a role in the disease.

REFERENCES

1. **Hurst, A. F.,** Ulcerative colitis, *Guys Hosp. Rep.,* 71, 26, 1921.
2. **Onderdonk, A. B. and Bartlett, J. G.,** Bacteriological studies of experimental ulcerative colitis, *Am. J. Clin. Nutr.,* 32, 258, 1979.
3. **Van der Waaij, D., Cohen, B. J., and Anver, M. R.,** Mitigation of experimental inflammatory bowel disease in Guinea pigs by selective elimination of aerobic gram negative intestinal flora, *Gastroenterology,* 67, 460, 1974.
4. **Levine, M. M.,** *Escherichia coli* that cause diarrhoea: enterotoxigenic, enteropathogenic, enteroinvasive, enterohaemorrhagic, and enteroadherent, *J. Infect. Dis.,* 155, 377, 1987.
5. **Van de Weil-Korstanje, J. A. A. and Winkler, K. C.,** The faecal flora in ulcerative colitis, *J. Med. Microbiol.,* 8, 491, 1975.
6. **Gorbach, S. L., Nahas, L., Plaut, A. G., Weinstein, L., Patterson, J. F., and Levitan, R.,** Studies of intestinal microflora. V. Fecal microbial ecology in ulcerative colitis and regional enteritis: relationship to severity of disease and chemotherapy, *Gastroenterology,* 54, 575, 1968.
7. **Keighley, M. R. B., Arabi, Y., Dimck, F., Burdon, D. W., Allan, R. N., and Alexander-Williams, J.,** Influence of inflammatory bowel disease on intestinal microflora, *Gut,* 19, 1099, 1978.
8. **Cooke, E. M.,** A quantitative comparison of the faecal flora of patients with ulcerative colitis and that of normal persons, *J. Pathol. Bacteriol.,* 94, 439, 1967.
9. **Gorbach, S. L.,** Intestinal microflora, *Gastroenterology,* 60, 1110, 1971.
10. **Cooke, E. M.,** Properties of strains of *Escherichia coli* isolated from the faeces of patients with ulcerative colitis, patients with acute diarrhoea, and normal persons, *J. Pathol. Bacteriol.,* 95, 101, 1968.

11. **Cooke, E. M., Ewins, S., Hywell-Jones, J., and Lennard-Jones, J. E.,** Properties of strains of *Escherichia coli* carried in different phases of ulcerative colitis, *Gut*, 15, 143, 1974.

12. **Tabaqchali, S., O'Donoghue, D. P., and Bettelheim, K. A.,** *Escherichia coli* antibodies in patients with inflammatory bowel disease, *Gut*, 19, 108, 1978.

13. **Lagercrantz, R., Hammarstrom, S., Perlamann, P., and Gustafsson, B. E.,** Immunological studies in ulcerative colitis. IV. Origin of autoantibodies, *J. Exp. Med.*, 128, 1339, 1968.

14. **Kemler, B. J. and Alpert, E.,** Inflammatory bowel disease: study of cell-mediated cytotoxicity for isolated colonic epithelial cells, *Gut*, 21, 353, 1980.

15. **Smith, H. W. and Linggood, Ma.,** Observations on the pathogenic properties of the K88, Hly and Ent plasmids of *Escherichia coli* with particular reference to porcine diarrhoea, *J. Med. Microbiol.*, 4, 467, 1971.

16. **Satterwhite, T. K., Evans, D. G., Dupont, H. L., and Evans, D. J., Jr.,** Role of *Escherichia coli* colonisation factor antigen in acute diarrhoea, *Lancet*, ii, 181, 1978.

17. **Levine, M. M., Nataro, J. P., Karch, H., et al.** The diarrhoeal response of humans to some classical serotypes of enteropathogenic *Escherichia coli* is dependant on a plasmid encoding an enteroadhesive factor, *J. Infect. Dis.*, 152, 550, 1985.

18. **Orskov, F. and Orskov, I.,** Serotyping of *Escherichia coli*, *Methods Microbiol.*, 14, 44, 1984.

19. **Duguid, J. P., Clegg, S., and Wilson, M. I.,** The fimbrial and non-fimbrial haemagglutinins of *Escherichia coli*, *J. Med. Microbiol.*, 12, 2, 1979.

20. **Evans, D. J., Jr., Evans, D. G., Youn, L. S., and Pitt, J.,** Haemagglutination typing of *Escherichia coli*: Definition of seven haemagglutination types, *J. Microbiol.*, 12, 235, 1980.

21. **Evans, D. G. and Evans, D. J.,** New surface-associated heat-labile colonization factor antigen (CFA/II) produced by enterotoxigenic *Escherichia coli* of serogroups 06 and 08, *Infect. Immun.*, 12, 656, 1975.

22. **Penaranda, M. E., Mann, M. B., and Evans, D. J.,** Transfer of an ST: LT: CFA/II plasmid into *Escherichia coli* K-12 strain RRI by cotransformation with pSC301 plasmid DNA, *FEMS Microbiol. Lett.*, 8, 251, 1980.

23. **Parry, S. H. and Rooke, D. M.,** Adhesins and colonisation factors, in *The Virulence of Escherichia coli. Reviews and Methods*. Sussman, M., Ed., Academic Press, London, 1985, 79.

24. **Dickinson, F. J., Varian, S. A., Axon, A. T. R., and Cooke, E. M.,** Increased incidence of faecal coliforms with *in vitro* adhesive and invasive properties in patients with ulcerative colitis, *Gut*, 21, 787, 1980.

25. **Ellen, R. P., Fillery, E. D., Chan, K. H., and Grove, D. A.,** Sialidase-enhanced lectin-like mechanism for *Actinomyces viscosus* and *Actinomyces naeslundii* haemagglutination, *Infect. Immun.*, 27, 335, 1980.

26. **Parsons, C. L., Shrom, S. H., Hanno, P. M., and Mulholland, S. G.,** Bladder surface mucin. Examination of possible mechanisms for its antibacterial effect, *Invest. Urol.*, 16, 196, 1978.

27. **Pinder, I. F., Dickinson, R. J., Cooke, E. M., and Axon, A. T. R.,** High incidence of potentially pathogenic *E. coli* in first attacks of idiopathic colitis, *Gut*, 24, A997, 1983.

28. **Jones, G. W. and Rutter, J. M.,** Role of the K-88 antigen in the pathogenesis of neonatal diarrhoea caused by *Escherichia coli* in piglets, *Infect. Immun.*, 6, 918, 1972.

29. **Rutter, J. M., Burrows, M. R., Dellwood, R., and Gibbons, R. A.,** A genetic basis for resistance to enteric disease caused by *E. coli*, *Nature*, 257, 135, 1975.

30. **Dickinson, R. J., Branch, W. J., Warren, R. E., and Neale, G.,** Rectal organ culture as a model for the investigation of bacterial adhesion and invasion, *J. Clin. Pathol.*, 37, 587, 1984.

31. **Burke, D. A. and Axon, A. T. R.,** Ulcerative colitis and *Escherichia coli* with adhesive properties, *J. Clin. Pathol.*, 40, 782, 1987.

32. **Challacombe, D. N., Richardson, J. M., Rowe, B., and Anderson, C. M.,** Bacterial microflora of the upper gastrointestinal tract in infants with protracted diarrhoea, *Arch. Dis. Child.*, 49, 270, 1974.

33. **Candy, D. C. A., Leung, T. S. M., Philips, A. D., Harries, J. T., and Marshall, W. C.,** Models for studying the adhesion of enterobacteria to the mucosa of the human intestinal tract, in *Adhesion and Microorganism Pathogenicity*, Elliot, K. and O'Connor, J., Eds., Pittman Medical, Tunbridge Wells, 1981, 72.

34. **Burke, D. A. and Axon, A. T. R.,** HeLa and buccal epithelial cell adhesion assays for detecting intestinal *Escherichia coli* with adhesive properties in ulcerative colitis, *J. Clin. Pathol.*, 40, 1402, 1987.

35. **Burke, D. A. and Axon, A. T. R.,** Adhesive *Escherichia coli* in inflammatory bowel disease and infective diarrhoea, *Br. Med. J.*, 297, 102, 1988.

36. **Lane, M. R., Allan, R. N., and Pease, P. E.,** Antibiotic resistance in *Escherichia coli* from patients on sulfasalazine, *Lancet*, 1, 1403, 1988.

37. **Burke, D. A., Clayden, S. A., and Axon, A. T. R.,** Sulfasalazine does not select for *Escherichia coli* with adhesive properties in ulcerative colitis, *Lancet*, ii, 966, 1988.

38. **Jones, G. W.,** The attachment of bacteria to the surfaces of animal cells, in *Microbial Interactions, Receptors and Recognition, Ser. B*, Reissig, J. L., Chapman and Hall, London, 1977, 139.

39. **Lindahl, M., Faris, A., Wadstrom, T., and Hjerten, S.,** A new test based on salting out to measure relative surface hydrophobicity of bacterial cells, *Biochem. Biophys. Acta*, 677, 471, 1981.

40. **Burke, D. A. and Axon, A. T. R.,** Hydrophobic adhesin of *E. coli* in ulcerative colitis, *Gut*, 29, 41, 1988.

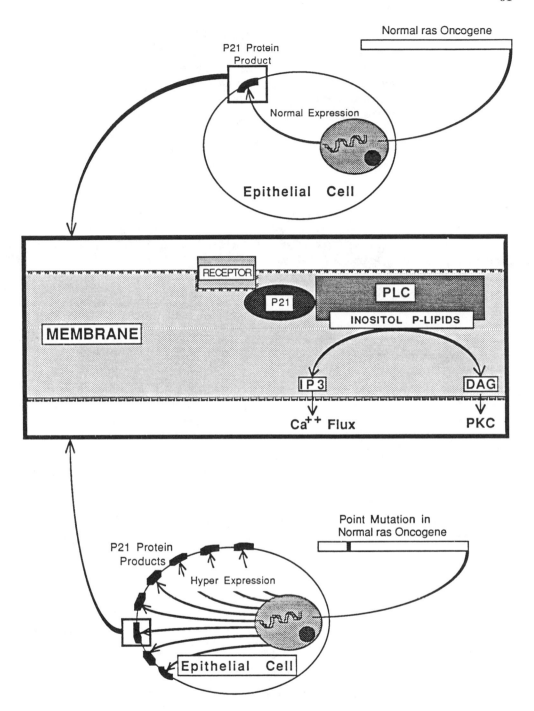

FIGURE 2. Function the of *ras* oncogenes and their p21 protein product. p21 protein product produced by *ras* oncogene appears to link against receptor interaction to phospholipase C (PLC) activation. PLC catalyzes the hydrolysis of inositol phospholipids to generate inositol tris-phosphate (IP3) and diacyl glyceral (DAG). These second messengers are involved in the regulation of cell growth and proliferation through their effects on calcium flux and protein kinase C activation, respectively. The lower half of the panel demonstrates the effect of a point mutation in a *ras* oncogene resulting in uncontrolled production of p21 protein product with potential amplification of activation of PLC.

An alternative group of genes, the so called antioncogenes, has been reported. These genes, which code for putative regulatory products, are present in normal individuals; however, their expression is reduced or abberant in specific neoplasia such as retinoblastoma and Wilm's tumor.[55,56] Linkage studies have located the gene for the familial adenomatous polyposis gene on chromosome 5q. Further studies performed, using a minisatellite probe, demonstrated that at least 20% of individuals with colonic carcinoma demonstrate chromosome 5 allele loss. With distinction to the genes involved in the development of retinoblastoma, deletion of a single allele appears to be associated with malignancy. Such studies have not as yet been extended to ulcerative colitis. However, it is conceivable that patients with UC who go on to develop carcinoma show similar allele loss. Allelic deletions of chromosome 17 and 18 also occur in approximately 75% of cases of colonic carcinoma.[57] However, while chromosome 18 loss occurred both in colonic carcinomas and adenomas, chromosome 17 was lost only in cases of carcinoma. The recent suggestion that a number of mutations, including mutations involved in increasing quantities of oncogene products and mutations in genes with antionco-gene or tumor-repressor properties, may be necessary for the development of colonic cancer suggests a complex regulatory system for growth and proliferation of colonic epithelial cells which is currently poorly understood. Thus, it is critically important to determine whether allelic deletions also occur in chromosomes 5, 17, and 18 in ulcerative colitis.

VI. CONCLUSIONS

Techniques in molecular biology provide a potent tool in the analysis of disease pathogenesis. Thus far, there is a small but important body of research in inflammatory bowel disease resulting from these techniques. The potential applications of molecular biology to the study of ulcerative colitis are extremely wide. Areas ranging from genetics to the search for a potential infective agent can be explored.

ACKNOWLEDGMENT

The author wishes to thank P. Curtis Mazur for preparation of the figures and Dr. Bruce Torbett for critical review of the manuscript.

REFERENCES

1. **Beam, K. G.,** Duchenne muscular dystrophy. Localizing the gene product [news], *Nature,* 33, 798, 1988.
2. **Williamson, R., Wainwright, B., Cooper, C., Scambler, P., Farrall, M., Estivill, X., and Pedersen, P.,** The cystic fibrosis locus (Review), *Enzyme,* 38, 8, 1987.
3. **Omata, M., Yokosuka, O., Imazeki, F., et al.,** Correlation of hepatitis B virus DNA and antigens in the liver, *Gastroenterology,* 92, 192, 1987.
4. **Marcussen, H. and Nerup, J.,** Fluorescent anti-colon and organ specific antibodies in ulcerative colitis, *Scand. J. Gastroenterol.,* 8, 9, 1973.
5. **Shorter, R. G., McGill, D. B., and Bahn, R. C.,** Cytotoxicity of mononuclear cells for autologous colonic epithelial cells in colonic disease, *Gastroenterology,* 86, 13, 1984.
6. **Kelleher, D., Murphy, A., Feighery, C., Whelan, C. A., Kelling, P. W. N., and Weir, D. G.,** Defective suppression in the AMLR in patients with Crohn's disease, *Gut,* 30, 839, 1989.
7. **Sanz, I. and Capra, J. D.,** The genetic origin of human autoantibodies, *J. Immunol.,* 140, 3283, 1988.
8. **Zanetti, M., Glotz, D., and Sollazzo, M.,** Idiotype regulation of self responses, autoantibody V regions and neonatal B Cell repertoire, *Immunol. Lett.,* 16, 277, 1987.
9. **Bona, C. A.,** V genes encoding autoantibodies: molecular and phenotypic characteristics, *Annu. Rev. Immunol.,* 6, 327, 1988.

10. **Kasturi, K., Monestier, M., Mayer, R., and Bona, C.,** Biased usage of certain Vk gene families by autoantibodies and their polymorphism in autoimmune mice, *Mol. Immunol.,* 213, 1988.

11. **Kagnoff, M. F., Brown, R. J., and Schanfield, M. S.,** Association between Crohn's disease and immuno-globulin heavy chain (Gm) allotypes, *Gastroenterology,* 85, 1044, 1983.

12. **Ghanem, N., Dugoujon, J. M., Bensmana, M., Huck, S., Lefranc, M. P., and Lefranc, G.,** Restriction fragment haplotypes in the human immunoglobulin IGHG locus and their correlation with the Gm polymorphism, *Eur. J. Immunol.,* 18, 1067, 1988.

13. **Davis, M. M. and Bjorkman, P. J.,** T-cell receptor genes and T-cell recognition, *Nature,* 334, 335, 1988.

14. **Volk, B. A., Howell, M. D., Smith, J., and Kagnoff, M. F.,** Association of a polymorphic human T-cell receptor a chain fragment with ulcerative colitis, *Gastroenterology,* 94, A482, 1988.

15. **Todd, J. A., Bell, J. I., and McDevitt, O.,** HLA-DQ beta gene contributes to susceptibility and resistance to insulin-dependent diabetes mellitus, *Nature,* 329, 599, 1987.

16. **Sinha, A. A., Brautbar, C., Szafer, F., Friedmann, A., Tzfoni, E., Todd, J. A., Steinman, L., and McDevitt, H. Q.,** A newly characterized HLA DQ beta allele associated with pemphigus vulgaris, *Science,* 239, 1026, 1988.

17. **Nepom, G. T., Hansen, J. A., and Nepom, B. S.,** The molecular basis for HLA class II associations with rheumatoid arthritis, *J. Clin. Immunol.,* 7, 1, 1987.

18. **Carroll, M. C., Katzman, P., Alicot, E. M., Koller, B. H., Geraghty, D. E., Orr, H. T., Strominger, J. L., and Spies, T.,** Linkage map of the human major histocompatibility complex including the tumor necrosis factor genes, *Proc. Natl. Acad. Sci. U.S.A.,* 84(23), 8535, 1987.

19. **Sanchez Perez, M. and Shaw, S.,** *Human Class II Histocompatibility Antigens: Theoretical and Practical Aspects,* Springer-Verlag, New York, p. 83.

20. **Ando, A., Inoko, H., Kimura, M., Ogata, S., and Tsuji, K.,** Isolation and allelic polymorphism of cDNA clones and genomic clones of HLA-DP heavy and light chains, *Hum. Immunol.,* 17, 355, 1986.

21. **Howell, M. D., Smith, J. R., Austin, R. K., Kelleher, D., Nepom, G. T., Volk, B., and Kagnoff, M. F.,** An extended HLA-D region haplotype associated with celiac disease, *Proc. Natl. Acad. Sci. U.S.A.,* 85, 222, 1988.

22. **Delpre, G., Kadish, U., Gazit, E., Joshua, H., and Zamir, R.,** HLA antigens in ulcerative colitis and Crohn's disease in Israel, *Gastroenterology,* 78, 1452, 1980.

23. **Miyamoto, K., Ishii, H., Takata, H., et al.,** Association of HLA-B40 and DRw9 with Japanese alcoholic liver cirrhosis, *Pharmacol. Biochem. Behav.,* 18 (Suppl. 1.1), 467, 1983.

24. **Asakura, H., Tsuchiya, M., Aiso, S., et al.,** Association of the human lymphocyte DR2 antigen with Japanese ulcerative colitis, *Gastroenterology,* 82, 413, 1982.

25. **Kobayashi, K., Sekiguchi, S., Ato, M., Inoko, H., Yagit, A., and Tsuji, K.,** Southern blot analysis of HLA class II beta gene in Crohn's disease, presented at the 6th Int. Congr. of Immunol., Toronto, Canada, 1986.

26. **Ness, D. B. and Grumet, F. C.,** New polymorphisms of HLA-B27 and other B Locus antigens detected by RFLP using a locus-specific probe, *Hum. Immunol.,* 18, 65, 1987.

27. **Coppin, H. L. and McDevitt, H. O.,** Absence of polymorphisms between HLA-B27 genomic exon sequences isolated from normal donors and ankylosing spondylitis patients, *J. Immunol.,* 137, 2168, 1986.

28. **Bodmer, W. F., Bailey, C. J., Bodmer, J., et al.,** Localisation of the gene for familial adenomatous polyposis on chromosome 5, *Nature,* 328, 614, 1987.

29. **Cannon-Albright, L. A., Skolnick, M. H., Bishop, D. T., Lee, R. G., and Burt, R. W.,** Common inheritance of susceptibility to colonic adenomatous polyps and associated colorectal cancers, *N. Engl. J. Med.,* 319, 533, 1988.

30. **Lotz, M., Carson, D. A., and Vaughan, J. H.,** Substance P activation of rheumatoid synoviocytes: a neural pathway in pathogenesis of arthritis, *Science,* 803, 1987.

31. **Mantyh, C. R., Gates, T. S., Zimmerman, et al.,** Receptor binding sites for substance P but not substance K or neuromedin K are expressed in high concentrations by arterioles, venules and lymph nodules in surgical specimens obtained from patients with ulcerative colitis and Crohn's disease, *Proc. Natl. Acad. Sci. U.S.A.,* 85, 3235, 1988.

32. **Weinstock, J. V., Blum, A., Walder, J., and Walder, R.,** Eosinophils from granulomas in murine *Schisto-miasis mansoni* produce substance P, *J. Immunol.,* 141, 961, 1988.

33. **Zeitz, M., Greene, W. C., Peffer, N. J., and James, S. P.,** Lymphocytes isolated from the intestinal lamina propria of normal nonhuman primates have increased expression of genes associated with T-cell activation, *Gastroenterology,* 94, 647, 1988.

34. **Volk, B. A., Kelleher, D., Harwood, J., Brenner, D. A., and Kagnoff, M. F.,** Comparison of HLA class II transcripts in human small intestinal biopsies, *Gastroenterology,* 94, A482, 1988.

35. **Rappolee, D. A., Mark, D., Banda, M. J., and Werb, Z.,** Wound macrophages express TGF-alpha and other growth factors *in vivo:* analysis by MRNA phenotyping, *Science,* 241, 708, 1988.

36. **Kaulfersch, W., Fiocchi, C., and Waldmann, T. A.,** Polyclonal nature of the intestinal mucosal lymphocyte populations in inflammatory bowel disease, *Gastroenterology,* 95, 364, 1988.

37. **Mullis, K., Falloona, F., Scharf, S., Saiki, R., Horn, G., and Erlich, H.,** Specific enzymatic amplification of DNA *in vitro:* the polymerase chain reaction, *Cold Spring Harbor Symp. Quant. Biol.,* 51(Part 1), 263, 1986.

38. **Roche, J. K., Wold, W. S. M., Sander, P. R., Mackey, J. K., and Green, M.,** Chronic inflammatory bowel disease: absence of adenovirus DNA as established by molecular hybridisation, *Gastroenterology,* 81, 853, 1981.

39. **Chiodine, R. J., Van Kreuningen, H. J., Thayer, W. R., Merkal, R. S., and Contu, J.,** The possible role of mycobacteria in inflammatory bowel disease — an unclassified *Mycobacterium* species isolated from patients with Crohn's disease, *Dig. Dis. Sci.,* 29, 1073, 1984.

40. **McFadden, J. J., Butcher, P. D., Chiodine, R., and Hermon-Taylor, J.,** Crohn's disease-isolated mycobacteria are identical to *Mycobacterium paratuberculosis* as determined by DNA probes that distinguish between mycobacterial species, *J. Clin. Microbiol.,* 25, 796, 1987.

41. **Whitman, M., Fleischman, L., Chahwals, S. B., Cantley, L., and Rosoff, P.,** Phosphoinositides, mitogenesis and oncogenesis, in *Phosphoinositides and Rectotor Mechanisms,* Alan R. Liss, New York, 1986, 197.

42. **Eisenman, R. N. and Thompson, C. B.,** Oncogenes with potential nuclear function, *Cancer Surv.,* 5, 309, 1986.

43. **Wakelam, M. J., Davies, S. A., Houslay, M. D., McKay, M. D., Marshall, C. J.,and Hall, A.,** Normal p21 N-ras couples bombesin and other growth factors to inositol phosphate hydrolysis, *Nature,* 323, 173, 1986.

44. **Capon, D. J., Chen, E. Y., Levinson, A. D., Seeburg, P. H., and Goeddel, D. V.,** Complete nucleotide sequence of the T24 human bladder carcinoma oncogene and its normal homologue, *Nature,* 302, 33, 1983.

45. **Bos, J. L., Fearon, E. R., Hamilton, S. R., et al.,** Prevalence of ras gene mutations in human colorectal cancers, *Nature,* 327, 293, 1987.

46. **Forrester, K., Almoguera, C., Han, K., Grizzle, W. E., and Perucho, M.,** Detection of high incidence of K-ras oncogenes during human colon tumorigenesis, *Nature,* 327, 298, 1987.

47. **Michelassi, F., Leuthner, S., Lubienski, M., et al.,** Ras oncogene p21 levels parallel malignant potential of different human colonic benign conditions, *Arch. Surg.,* 122, 1414, 1987.

48. **Meltzer, S. J.,** Oncogene expression in ulcerative colitis, *Gastroenterology,* 92, 1530, 1988.

49. **Meltzer, S. J. and Weinstein, W. M.,** Oncogene expression in Barrett's esophagus, *Gastroenterology,* 92, 1530, 1988.

50. **Ciclitera, P. J., Macartney, J. C., and Evan, G.,** Expression of C-*myc* in non-malignant and pre-malignant gastrointestinal disorders, *J. Pathol.,* 151, 293, 1987.

51. **Collins, J. F., Damm, D., and Bagby, G. C.,** Increased expression of Ha-ras colon of rats with carcinogen induced colorectal carcinoma, *Gastroenterology,* 92, 1352, 1987.

52. **Quintanilla, M., Brown, K., Ramsden, M., and Balmain, A.,** Carcinogen specific mutation and amplification of Ha-ras during mouse skin carcinogenesis, *Nature,* 322, 78, 1986.

53. **Cohen, J. B. and Levinson, A. D.,** A point mutation in the las intron responsible for increased expression and transforming activity of c-Ha-ras oncogene, *Nature,* 334, 119, 1988.

54. **Nishizuka, Y.,** The role of protein kanase C in cell surface signal transduction and tumor promotion, *Nature,* 308, 693, 1984.

55. **Whyte, P., Buchkovich, K. J., Horowitz, J. M., et al.,** Association between an oncogene and an anti-oncogene: the adenovirus E1A proteins bind to the retinoblastoma gene product, *Nature,* 334, 124, 1988.

56. **Davis, L. M., Stallard, R., Thomas, G. H., et al.,** Two anonymous DNA segments distinguish the Wilm's tumour and Aniridia loci, *Science,* 241, 840, 1988.

57. **Vogelstein, B., Fearon, E. R., Hamilton, S. R., et al.,** Genetic alterations during colorectal-tumour development, *N. Engl. J. Med.,* 319, 525, 1988.

Chapter 7

COLONIC MUCUS AND ULCERATIVE COLITIS

G. F. Cope, R. V. Heatley, and J. Kelleher

TABLE OF CONTENTS

I. GENERAL INTRODUCTION

The colonic mucosal defenses have been extensively investigated as to whether they may have a role in the etiology and pathogenesis of ulcerative colitis. Although many abnormalities have been detected, the colonic mucus layer appears to be consistently abnormal. Studies have shown qualitative and quantitative changes, which suggests that it does not possess the physical characteristics to provide complete epithelial protection.[1-3]

Mucus is an intricate viscoelastic gel which forms a continuous protective layer over the entire epithelial surface of the gastrointestinal tract.[4-6] The actual thickness is variable, not only between different regions of the gastrointestinal tract, but also within an individual section of mucosa.[7] The mucus layer is a dynamic entity, with the overall thickness depending upon the amount of mucus produced and the degree of degradation due to proteolytic digestion and erosion by shear forces. Studies have shown that the colonic mucus layer is approximately 200 μm in thickness, with a range of 5 to 350 μm (Cope, unpublished data), which is comparable with data obtained for gastric mucus.[7]

Mucus is a complex secretion which has evolved to play an active role in the protection of the mucosal surface.[8] The primary function of gastrointestinal mucus is thought to be the protection of the underlying epithelial cells from mechanical damage, by lubricating the passage of food or feces, and the biochemical process of digestion. It can withstand osmotic changes and is sufficiently fluid to resist physical disruption, allowing it to flow into and heal breakages.[6] Mucus also serves as a selectively permeable barrier preventing large, potentially harmful substances including antigens, toxins, and enzymes from making contact with the mucosa by means of a process known as polymer exclusion.[9] Mucus also acts as a physical support for other epithelial secretions, including lysozyme, lactoferrin, and secretory IgA, and is also capable of adhering to and engulfing unicellular and multicellular organisms facilitating their expulsion by peristalsis.[8]

II. MUCUS STRUCTURE

Gastrointestinal mucus is a complex mixture, consisting mainly of water (approximately 95% by weight), and containing various serum and cellular macromolecules, electrolytes, microorganisms, and sloughed cells.[10] It possesses the structure and physical properties of a true gel, due to the presence of a network of cross-linked polymers called mucus glycoproteins.[11] These form an expanded, entangled, unstirred matrix immersed in water, the configuration of which is such that it can exist in two distance phases — a viscous insoluble adherent gel and a soluble nonadherent liquid sol.

Mucus glycoproteins are extremely large molecular weight components and are rich in carbohydrate, which accounts for up to 85% of the glycoprotein by weight. The molecular structure of the glycoproteins consist of a central protein core rich in the amino acids serine, threonine, and, to a lesser extent, proline. The first two serve as attachment points for the carbohydrate polymers (oligosaccharides) which are joined via an alpha linkage to the hydroxyl oxygen of the amino acid, forming an O-glycosidic linkage.[12] The oligosaccharide chains vary in length from 2 to about 20 sugar residues, and they can be linear or branched. The oligosaccharides are extremely numerous and heterogeneous. One estimate puts the number of oligosaccharide units in colonic mucus glycoprotein molecules at approximately 3000 units, all with the potential for almost unlimited structural polydispersity.[8] They are formed, however, from only five monosaccharide residues: galactose (Gal), *N*-acetylglucosamine (GlcNac), *N*-acetylgalactosamine (GalNac), *N*-acetylneuraminic acid (NeuNac) — commonly known as sialic acid, and fucose (Fuc). Mucus glycoproteins can also undergo sulfate substitution at the point of GalNac and Gal residues (Figure 1).

The initial link between the protein core and the oligosaccharide chain is always via a

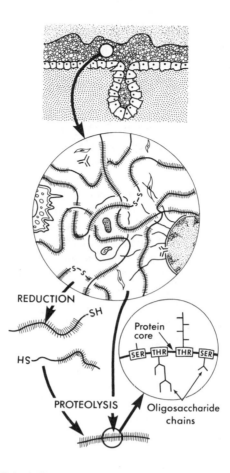

FIGURE 1. A diagram of colonic mucus which is depicted as a layer of variable thickness over the entire epithelial surface. Mucus is an aqueous mixture of microorganisms, sloughed cells, immunoglobulins, and serum and cellular macromolecules, the most important of which are the "bottle brush"-like mucus glycoproteins. These form an entangled network of cross-linked polymers linked together by disulfide bridges. Reduction of mucus results in the unlinking of the disulfide bonds producing glycoprotein "subunits". Proteolysis attacks the "naked areas" of the glycoprotein, producing mucin glycopeptides. Mucus glycoproteins consist of a central protein core to which is attached, at the point of serine or threonine residues, numerous heterogeneous oligosaccharide chains.

GalNac unit. Generally, subsequent sugar residues are added via beta linkages in a variety of combinations which appear to be modifications of specific repeating sequences. Despite this, the number of different combinations that can be achieved within one glycoprotein molecule is extremely large. This variation of oligosaccharides is in marked contrast to the protein core which is remarkably similar in all molecules of a specific glycoprotein.

The structural diversity of the carbohydrate moieties of glycoproteins is believed to provide the means for molecular recognition, which is particularly important in intercellular interactions. Specific terminal sugar residues are responsible for producing antigenic blood grouping determinants, such as in the ABO system.[13] The same terminal sugars are present in mucus glycoproteins, and consequently mucus can exhibit blood group characteristics.

Although the major part of the protein core of mucus glycoproteins is glycosylated, there are terminal sections, rich in aspartic acid, glutamic acid, valine, glycine, and alanine, which remain exposed, and these are referred to as "naked areas". These terminal sites enable different glycoprotein molecules or "subunits" to link together or polymerize, usually by means of covalent disulfide bridges. Evidence suggests however that such linkages are significantly less important in colonic mucus than in gastric mucus glycoproteins[14,16] and the existence of nonglycosylated domains within colonic mucin peptides has not yet been demonstrated.[16]

Work by Allen et al. on pig gastric mucus has indicated that on average four glycoprotein "subunits" were linked together to form a three-dimensional "windmill-like" configuration, with a resultant molecular weight of 2×10^6 Da.[17,18] More recent evidence by Carlstedt and Sheehan however has suggested an alternative model in which the glycoprotein subunits are long polypeptides with glycosylated and naked regions. The whole glycoprotein polymer forms a longer, linear, partially coiled thread with the unglycosylated regions being flexible and convoluted. The three dimensional structure is a spherical, hydrodynamic domain in solution.[12,19] Carlstedt suggests that this model more closely fits the available physicochemical data. Electron microscopic evidence supports the theory that the glycoprotein polymers are threads and not star-shaped tetramers, as previously suggested.[20] However, neither of these models is totally compatible with all of the available information; therefore, the conformation and molecular size of mucus glycoproteins still remains a matter of controversy.[21]

Purified mucus glycoproteins have been found to contain significant quantities of noncovalently bound protein and lipid which are attached to the naked regions of the glycoproteins.[21,23] These are thought to protect the unglycosylated regions from proteolytic attack[24,25] and their removal generally results in a weaker gel formation.

III. MUCUS SECRETION

Production of gastrointestinal mucus occurs within the specialized goblet cells of the epithelium. These cells are a major component of the colonic epithelium, interdispersed with absorptive cells. They are also present within the epithelial crypts where they are intermingled with undifferentiated proliferative cells and more specialized endocrine cells.[16]

The synthesis of mucus glycoproteins is initiated by the assembly of the protein core in the endoplasmic reticulum. This involves transcription from the genetic code, involving a number of structural genes. The polypeptides produced by a homogeneous goblet cell population will therefore be very similar, although regional variations will occur.[26] Glycosylation of the protein commences in the endoplasmic reticulum and progresses in the Golgi apparatus.[27] The monosaccharide residues following activation to nucleotide sugars are transferred to the protein by membrane-bound substrate-specific glycotransferases.[28,29] The monosaccharides are then sequentially transferred to form the oligosaccharide chains.[12] Glycosylation is initiated by the transfer of a GalNac residue to either serine or threonine and continues with the formation of an extended "backbone" or core region. Intestinal mucins only appear to contain two types of core region. Subsequent addition of monosaccharides can give rise to branching, either distal or proximal to the polypeptide, according to which sequence of sugars is produced. The later stages of glycosylation, when the terminal sugars are attached, is performed in the trans-Golgi apparatus. The presence of GalNac and Gal groups allows for substitution with either sulfate group and it is the sulfate groups together with the NeuNac groups which are largely responsible for the polyionic character of the glycoproteins.[12,27] These groups are particularly important in colonic mucus glycoproteins.

The completed glycoprotein molecule will probably undergo tertiary transformations in three dimensions due to ionic interactions between the sugars and amino acids and will also polymerize by means of disulfide bond formation.[30,31] The completed glycoprotein molecules are stored within membrane-bound granules which congregate in the apical regions of the cell. The mature granules are relatively uniform in size and do not perceptibly change as they move toward the cell surface.[10]

The control of intestinal mucus release was investigated by Florey in the 1930s. He suggested that secretion was stimulated by "...mechanical, thermal and chemical insult coming from the lumen of the intestine."[32] His investigations led to our understanding of the importance of the autonomic nervous system in the general control of mucus secretion. Local stimuli however appear capable of initiating mucus release independent of neuronal involvement, but only in the immediate vicinity of the stimulus.[33,34] The modern view of intestinal mucus secretion is that it functions on three levels. First, there is the slow, continuous replenishment of the mucus layer from the epithelial surface to compensate for loss and destruction at the luminal surface. This is believed to occur spontaneously, with discharge of small quantities of stored goblet cell contents. Second, there is systemic control which modifies intestinal mucus secretion according to homeostatic needs,[35] which is controlled by the autonomic and enteric nervous systems. Third, there is the rapid, almost explosive, release of mucus which follows local irritation and forms an "emergency" blanket of mucus which protects the mucosa at times of potential damage.[36]

Studies of mucus production have shown that secretion, but not synthesis, is under the control of the cholinergic parasympathetic nervous system, responding to both endogenous and exogenous muscarinic-type agonists such as acetylcholine, pilocarpine, and carbachol, the effects of which can be blocked by atropine.[37–40] The role of the sympathetic nervous system is, however, less certain. Intestinal mucus secretion has been stimulated by the beta adrenergic agonist isoprenaline;[39,41] however, subsequent investigations have failed to show any stimulatory effect.[35,37,42] The nonadrenergic, noncholinergic inhibitory nerves which form part of the intrinsic nervous system are believed to play an important role in intestinal mucus secretion. Neuronal peptides such as vasoactive intestinal peptide; substance P and the purine nucleotides, such as ATP or adenosine, have been investigated, but their true effects are as yet unclear. Histamine and 5-HT have also been found to stimulate large intestinal mucus secretion *in vitro,* an effect which is independent of the parasympathetic nervous system.[37,40]

The goblet cells which are sensitive to neuronal stimulation are the immature cells which remain at the base of the epithelial crypts, the mature cells at the epithelial surface are insensitive.[36,43] It seems that as the immature cells migrate up the crypt sides they lose their responsiveness to neuronal mediators, possibly by loss or masking of the basolateral receptors. However, as they mature they develop an increased susceptibility to irritants. It is these cells which supply the bulk of the mucus layer under normal resting conditions.[44] Mucus production may also be influenced by conditions and agents which modify the differentiation and/ or migration of cells from the crypt to the epithelial surface.[16]

The inflammatory reaction was recognized by Florey as an important mediator of mucus secretion.[32] This has since been confirmed using inflammatory agents, such as the eicosanoids, which generally increase mucus production.[45,46] Alternatively, compounds such as the nonsteroidal antiinflammatory drugs which inhibit the inflammatory reaction have been shown to reduce mucus biosynthesis under certain conditions.[47] Cell-mediated immune responses also play a role in mucus secretion. Exposure of the intestinal mucosa to antigen-antibody immune complexes have been found to stimulate mucus release more than that stimulated by antigen absorption alone.[48] It appears that orally immunized animals have an enhanced response over those animals immunized by the i.v. route.[49] Other reports suggest that degranulation of mast cells, stimulated by an immune response, will also increase mucus release.[50]

The mechanisms by which mucus is released from the goblet cells was initially described as "an active process in which the droplets take up water and emerge through the free end of the cell, changing to fibers as they do so."[51] The actual mechanisms of mucus secretions appear to involve an orderly series of membrane fusion events in which mucus vesicles coalesce and then merge with the apical cell membrane, the granular contents being expelled by exocytosis. Recent evidence suggests that mucus is stored within the cell in a dehydrated state and only at the moment of release does it undergo a discontinuous phase transition when it hydrates and expands.[52] This involves Ca^{2+} and/or Cl^- ion interaction with the polyionic mucins, resulting in the final entangled glycoprotein network.[53.]

IV. MUCUS DEGRADATION

Although mucus glycoproteins are physically resistant to many aspects of physical and chemical disruption, they are susceptible to proteolytic and glycosidic degradation by enzymes produced by mucosal and bacterial cells. In the colon it is assumed that the endogenous flora secrete mucin proteases; however, this has not yet been confirmed.[10] However, colonic bacteria are known to release mucin-degrading glycosidases and sulfatases. The major site of colonic mucin degradation is the proximal colon, and this is the site of greatest bacterial accumulation.[54] Germ-free rats, which are devoid of colonic flora, excrete large quantities of mucins, which can be degraded by fecal bacteria from conventional rats.[55] Glyosidases capable of cleaving specific terminal sugars from the oligosaccharide chains are present in human fecal extracts and in the supernatant from anaerobic human fecal cultures.[55,56] Population studies estimate that mucin-degrading bacteria, which account for approximately five bacterial species, constitute 1% of the total colonic flora in healthy subjects.[56]

Bacterial mucin-degrading enzymes were first discovered by Hoskins et al;[57] a variety of substrate-specific mucin-degrading enzymes have now been described in fecal extracts.[58] Fortunately, colonic mucus has an inherent resistance to bacterial degradation probably afforded by the high concentrations of sulfate, NeuNac groups, and the presence of O-acyl NeuNac substitution.[59,60]

V. COLONIC MUCUS GLYCOPROTEINS IN HEALTH AND DISEASE

Histological staining techniques show normal healthy colonic mucus to be predominantly sialomucins and sulfomucins, with significant quantities of weakly staining neutral mucins.[61–63] This implies that the terminal residues of the oligosaccharide chains are mainly NeuNAc, sulfate, and Fuc, respectively. Regional variations have been detected in the types of mucins within the colon, with the relative amounts of sulfated mucins increasing distally along the colon, while the different forms of NeuNac group substitution, whether at the point of the C4, C7, and/or C8 atoms, also show regional differences.[64]

There also appear to be differences in the types of mucins within the epithelial crypts, with sialomucins being more abundant in the lower one third of the crypts, while sulfated mucins occupy the upper two thirds.[63,65] This suggests that as the cells mature and migrate up the crypt, their mucins either lose their sialic acid groups or else they are masked by the more dominant sulfated groups.[66] Acidic mucins can be subdivided according to their sensitivity to sialidase degradation. The majority of colonic mucins are sialidase resistant, probably due to the presence of O-acylated substitution on the NeuNac groups.[67]

Nonspecific inflammatory conditions of the colon are characterized by general reductions in total mucin compared with normal mucosa. In severely inflamed areas goblet cells can be reduced and sometimes almost completely absent. There may be a slight predominance of nonsulfated mucins, but otherwise there are no structural alterations either to the mucins or the colonic epithelium.[66]

Mucin depletion has long been recognized as a histological feature of ulcerative colitis. In mild disease there is a general reduction in the amount of mucus, with a relative increase in acidic, nonsulfated forms, probably caused by a loss of sulfated mucins and a deficiency of O-acetylated sialic acids associated with a decrease or total absence of neutral mucins.[67] In severe ulcerative colitis the mucin depletion is more evident and it appears to be related to disease severity.[63,68,69]

In contrast, the histochemical appearance of tissue from Crohn's disease shows that in most areas moderate to normal mucin secretion is maintained even in the presence of marked inflammation.[63] Histochemically, the mucins appear to be similar to normal, with perhaps a slight increase in nonsulfated mucins, but neutral mucins are generally present in normal amounts.[68,70]

Colonic carcinoma and the "transition zones" immediately surrounding a carcinoma have been found to have histochemical changes to their mucins. There is a gradual decrease in sulfated mucins in the lower crypts, with an equivalent increase in nonsulfated acidic mucins. Close to the tumor all acidic mucins are nonsulfated.[71]

Lectin-binding studies have proved useful in studying the structural characteristics of intestinal mucins. Such techniques have detected regional variations in colonic mucins,[72] as well as structural variations in inflammatory bowel disease. These findings generally substantiate the results obtained by histochemical techniques.[73,74]

In ulcerative colitis alterations to colonic mucus are accompanied by an increase in epithelial cell turnover. This is accompanied by crypt and epithelial distortion, with consequential reduction in goblet cell number.[67,73] These changes appear to be related to disease activity.[75-77] The replication of the cells is accompanied by exaggerated cell migration and premature exfoliation of epithelial cells. This implies that the cells are shed prematurely, before completing their normal cell cycle.[78] These changes can be demonstrated by scanning electron microscopy which shows that the normal colonic mucosa has an orderly array of closely packed circular crypts, the mouths of which are often stuffed with extruded mucus. The epithelium shows a "collar" of cells around the opening of the crypts, and the goblet cells are irregularly dispersed throughout. In chronic ulcerative colitis, with or without current inflammation, there is a reduction in the number of crypts, and those present are irregularly spaced and distorted. The epithelium undergoes structural alterations, forming furrows and cerebral-like ridges. These changes appear more pronounced where the tissue exhibits dysplasia.[79]

Biochemical analysis of colonic mucus by measurement of carbohydrate-containing material in mucosal biopsies was undertaken by Barton et al.[80] who showed that the sugar residues Fuc, Gas, GalNac, GluNac, NeuNac, and mannose (Mann) were present in approximately equal proportions. The overall composition was similar in both biopsy material and soluble luminal mucus.[80] Separation of the carbohydrate-containing material by liquid chromatography showed it to consist of two fractions of different molecular weight, the lower weight fractions containing mannose and the larger molecular weight being mannose-free. The presence of mannose was unusual because it is not a normal constituent of mucus glycoproteins. This mannose-containing material, evidently derived from secretory elements of the epithelium rather than from the plasma,[1] was found to be significantly increased in ulcerative colitis compared with normal. The large molecular weight material was decreased particularly in active disease.[3] The effects of this imbalance was that the larger mucus glycoproteins were diluted, with a resultant reduction in the viscosity of the mucus gel.[2] Further analysis showed that in ulcerative colitis there was an overall reduction in the amount of total carbohydrate in both the large and small molecular weight fractions, which appeared to be related to disease activity. Estimates of the average number of sugar residues in each oligosaccharide chain showed a reduction in ulcerative colitis to five from the normal of eight.[1] There was also a relative reduction in the quantities of serine and threonine in the protein core.[81]

Purification and isolation of colonic mucus glycoproteins from the pig by Marshall and Allen demonstrated the molecular weight to be 15×10^6 Da, and the isolated glycoproteins were considerable to be of a uniform molecular type.[15] LaMont and Ventola, using rat colonic mucus, also isolated an apparently homologous molecule, but further separation by ion-exchange chromatography showed it to consist of at least six separate peaks. Analysis of the sugar residues and amino acid content however showed that only two of the six peaks fulfilled the criteria of mucus glycoproteins, the remainder probably representing structural glycoproteins and mucus glycoprotein intermediates.[82] A similar procedure was used by Podolsky and Isselbacher to study possible structural alterations to colonic mucus in ulcerative colitis. Using resected colonic samples, adherent mucus was isolated and purified by means of gel filtration, nucleotide digestion, gradient centrifugation, and ion-exchange chromatography. The final separation revealed six peaks, all of which apparently satisfied the requirement for mucus glycoproteins. Two of the small fractions however were shown to contain mannose, albeit in minimal quantities.[83]

Analysis of material from patients with Crohn's disease and ischemic and infective colitis[83,84] showed no differences compared to normal. In ulcerative colitis however there was an overall reduction in the quantities of purified mucus, and ion-exchange chromatography revealed that one of the six mucin species, fraction IV, was consistently and dramatically reduced. This fraction accounted for approximately 15% of normal colonic mucus and was rich in sulfate and sialic acid residues. The reduction of fraction IV was seen in both active and inactive disease.[83]

Similar structural changes have been found in the colonic mucus of the cotton top tamarin (*Sanquinus oedipus*), a New World monkey which experiences a spontaneous relapsing colitis resembling idiopathic inflammatory bowel disease in humans.[16]

Using a modification of the original method, Podolsky studied mucus glycoproteins in biopsy samples and showed that, in addition to the deficiency in fraction IV, there were independent changes in fractions III and V which appeared to be restricted to inactive disease, disappearing when the disease was in relapse.[84]

Podolsky further analyzed the sequence of sugar residues in the oligosaccharide chains of the separate mucin subspecies. He confirmed the work of Slomiany[85] and showed that the chain length varied from 2 to 12 residues, and of the 21 different oligosaccharide structures identified, 10 were acidic and 11 were neutral in character. Many of the chains were common to a number of mucin species, yet some were restricted to a single subspecies. The results indicated that human colonic mucin contained a wide range of oligosaccharides reflecting variations of common core oligosaccharide structures.[86] Monoclonal antibodies were subsequently raised to the six separate human colonic mucus glycoproteins; from patterns of selective binding it became clear that both shared and species-specific antigenic determinants were present in the different mucin species.[87] Synthesis of the various glycoprotein types appeared to be by discrete goblet cell subpopulations, each producing distinctive combinations of mucin subspecies.[87] The goblet cells responsible for synthesis of fraction IV were found to be in the highest concentration at distal sites of the colon. This suggested that the specific reduction in ulcerative colitis could be due to a reduction or dysfunction of a particular goblet cell subpopulation.[88]

Although these biochemical studies are of utmost importance to the study of colonic mucus in ulcerative colitis, it should be noted that the reported findings have only originated from one center, and others have failed to confirm them.[89]

The assessment of mucus production by the colon has been largely undertaken using organ culture techniques and incorporation of radiolabeled precursors into newly synthesized mucus glycoproteins, with the amount of incorporation representing total mucus production.[90,91] In 1974, MacDermot et al. developed this technique to measure colonic mucus production by the incorporation of (^{14}C) glucosamine in biopsies removed from the rabbit colon and human rectum and maintained for 24 h in culture.[90] The newly synthesized lipid-free glycoproteins were isolated by acid precipitation followed by acid and organic solvent extraction. Autoradiography after organ culture allowed mucus biosynthesis to be followed as the radiolabeled precursor passed through the different intracellular organelles. Mucus secretion was also studied by the inclusion of neuronal mediators, such as acetylcholine, into the culture medium.[90]

The results showed that (^{14}C) glucosamine incorporation was significantly increased in rectal biopsies from patients with locally active ulcerative colitis compared to normal volunteers.[90] A subsequent study by Burton and Anderson using colonic biopsies from patients with inflammatory bowel disease showed that these patients had a significantly reduced incorporation compared with noninflammatory bowel disease patients. This study, unlike the previous report, examined colonic material from patients with active disease, taken from areas of the colon devoid of any active inflammation.[92]

A more recent study in our own laboratory examined colonic mucus production by (^{3}H) glucosamine incorporation in colonic biopsies removed from uninvolved areas and found that patients with ulcerative colitis incorporated significantly less radiolabel compared with patients with a normal colonic mucosa. Mucus production was also significantly reduced when the disease was in remission. During relapse, total colonic mucus production increased, largely due to an increase in mucus secretion, to a value similar to those obtained in controls.[93] From this and previous data it is apparent that mucus production is deficient in ulcerative colitis during disease remission but increases in active disease. This interpretation is in accordance with histochemical and lectin-binding studies which also indicate an increase in colonic mucus proportionate to disease severity.[63,94]

Organ culture techniques have also been used by Smith and Podolsky to study the relative production of colonic mucus glycoprotein subspecies.[95] They found that there were significant differences in the quantities of the subspecies released into the culture medium and those retained within the biopsy tissue. This suggested that some of the mucin subspecies were differentially secreted, whereas others were retained within the intracellular pools. Radiolabeled precursors were also incorporated into the subspecies at different rates, again suggesting that some subspecies were synthesized and secreted at different rates. Although the subspecies IV was found to be deficient in material from patients with ulcerative colitis, it was found that the amounts secreted into the culture medium were similar to controls. This prompted the hypothesis that in ulcerative colitis subspecies IV is differentially secreted rather than retained within the mucosal tissue.[95]

Examination of some of the enzymes involved in colonic mucus biosynthesis has shown possible modifications which may go some way toward explaining the changes in colonic mucus production. Glucosamine synthetase, which catalyzes the synthesis of glucosamine, has been found to be elevated in patients recovering from acute attacks of ulcerative colitis, suggesting either higher rates of mucus secretion or enhanced rates of mucus synthesis. Interestingly, histologically normal tissue from patients with Crohn's disease has also been found to have elevated levels.[96] The synthetic step following glucosamine synthetase is N-acetylation of the glucosamine, and is catalyzed by the enzyme transacetylase. This enzyme activity has been found to be diseased in patients with inflammatory bowel disease. This reduction suggested a possible malfunction in the mucus glycoprotein synthetic pathway subsequent to glucosamine synthetase in patients with inflammatory bowel disease.[92]

Abnormal colonic mucus degradation has also been examined for a possible role in the etiology of inflammatory bowel disease. Glycosidic decomposition is the slow but gradual removal of the terminal sugars from the protective oligosaccharide chains which renders the protein core more vulnerable to proteolytic breakdown. Therefore, enhanced bacterial degradation due either to physically deficient mucus or else more active bacterial enzymes may contribute to excessive mucus breakdown and reduced colonic epithelial protection, thus increasing the risk of colonic disease.[58,59] Any attempt, however, to correlate specific mucus-degrading glycosidases with the presence of inflammatory bowel disease or its activity has failed to show any positive associations.[97–99] Fecal neuraminidase levels have been found to be increased during active ulcerative colitis;[100] lyases and proteases were also significantly different in patients with inflammatory bowel disease compared with normals.[99] This latter finding is significant since certain O-acyl substitutions of the NeuNac groups, which are thought to provide protection of the acidic groups, could be removed by these enzymes and so render colonic mucus in ulcerative colitics more vulnerable to bacterial degradation.[99]

The inflamed colonic mucosa associated with ulcerative colitis shows increased immunological activity, both humoral and cellular.[101] Local accumulation and activation of the cellular element of inflammation results in the release of toxic oxygen metabolites, lysosomal enzymes, and metabolites of arachidonic acid,[102] including prostaglandin (PG) E^2, leukotriene (LT) B^4, and 5-hydroxyeicosatetraenoic acid (5-HETE).[103-105] These products may contribute to the perpetuation of inflammation and result in tissue destruction.[102] Not only are these substances chemotactic, they are also potent stimulators of mucus secretion;[10,106] it may be that chronically elevated levels of these and similar inflammatory mediators result in colonic mucin depletion.

VI. ULCERATIVE COLITIS AND CIGARETTE SMOKING

A relatively recent discovery concerning the epidemiology of ulcerative colitis has provided a new approach for studying the etiology of the disease. It appears that current and previous smoking habits influence the onset and pathogenesis of this condition. Numerous epidemiological studies have shown that patients with ulcerative colitis tend to be "nonsmokers",[107-109] with only 12% of patients being "current smokers".[110] This is in contrast to patients with Crohn's disease, where 52% are current smokers, and to control groups where approximately 30% are current smokers.[109,111] This led to the proposal that smoking may protect against ulcerative colitis[112] and that a smoking habit may determine which type of inflammatory bowel disease develops in susceptible individuals.[111]

More recent studies however have also examined the effect of previous smoking habits on the onset of disease and the results are not quite so unequivocal. However, it does appear that "ex-smokers" are more common among patients with ulcerative colitis than in control groups and are at increased relative risk of the disease to either "never smokers" or current smokers.[113,114] The group with the highest relative risk is those who had stopped smoking for 4 years or more.[115]

In an attempt to discover a possible mechanism for these relationships we have examined the effects of current and previous smoking habits on colonic mucus production *in vitro*. We found that patients with ulcerative colitis who remained nonsmokers had a significantly reduced colonic mucus production compared with nonsmoking controls. Furthermore, in those patients who continued to smoke, mucus production increased, largely due to increased mucus secretion, relative to nonsmoking colitics, and reached a level that was approximately the same as that measured in all controls, irrespective of their current smoking habit. This suggested that smoking may help rectify a deficiency of mucus production in ulcerative colitis, by increasing the quantity and perhaps the quality of the mucus layer, while not appearing to influence production in the normal colon.[116]

The assessment of previous smoking habits on mucus production showed that in control patients mucus production was highest in never smokers, lower, but not significantly, in current smokers, and lower still in ex-smokers, with the difference reaching significance compared with never smokers. In the patients with ulcerative colitis the pattern appeared to be different, with current smokers having the highest mucus production, which progressively decreased in ex-smokers and never smokers.[117] These results suggest that cessation of smoking may disrupt the capacity of the normal colon for mucus production, which in turn reduces the mucosal defensive barrier, and may predispose to the onset of ulcerative colitis in susceptible individuals.

In summary, changes to the colonic mucus layer in ulcerative colitis are fundamental to the etiology of the disease; however, whether these changes are primary or secondary to inflammatory changes remains unclear. Further investigation is required on the characterization of the mucus glycoprotein structure, with the interaction of mucus production, inflammatory mediators, and mucus degradation being of primary importance. The effect of cigarette smoking on ulcerative colitis, and on colonic mucus in particular, may shed further light on what is an intriguing and complex problem.

REFERENCES

1. **Clamp, J. R.,** Gastrointestinal mucus, in *Recent Advances in Gastrointestinal Pathology,* Wright, R., Ed., W. B. Saunders, 1989, 47.
2. **Teague, R. H., Fraser, D., and Clamp, J. R.,** Changes in monosaccharide content of mucous glycoproteins in ulcerative colitis, *Br. Med. J.,* 2, 645, 1973.
3. **Clamp, J. R., Fraser, G., and Read, A. E.,** Study of the carbohydrate content of mucus glycoproteins from normal and diseased colons, *Clin. Sci.,* 61, 229, 1981.
4. **Clamp, J. R.,** The relationship between the immune system and mucus in the protection of mucous membranes, *Biochem. Soc. Trans.,* 12, 754, 1984.
5. **Allen, A.,** Mucus—a protective secretion of complexity, *TIBS,* 8, 169, 1983.
6. **Allen, A., Bell, A., Mantle, M., and Pearson, J. P.,** The structure and physiology of gastrointestinal mucus, *Adv. Exp. Med. Biol.,* 144, 115, 1982.
7. **Kerss, S., Allen, A., and Garner, A.,** A simple method for measuring thickness of the mucus gel layer adherent to rat, frog and human gastric mucosa: influence of feeding, prostaglandin, *N*-acetylcysteine and other agents, *Clin. Sci.,* 63, 187, 1982.
8. **Clamp, J.,** The role of mucus in human intestinal defense, in *Gut Defenses in Clinical Practice,* Losowsky, M. S. and Heatley, R. V., Eds., Churchill Livingstone, London, 1986, 83.
9. **Edwards, P. A. W.,** Is mucus a selective barrier to macromolecules?, *Br. Med. Bull.,* 34, 55, 1978.
10. **Neutra, M. R. and Forstner, J. F.,** Gastrointestinal mucus: synthesis, secretion, and function, in *Physiology of the Gastrointestinal Tract,* Johnson, L. R., Ed., Raven Press, New York, 1987, 975.
11. **Tanaka, T.,** Gels, *Sci. Am.,* 244, 110, 1981.
12. **Carlstedt, I., Sheehan, J. K., Corfield, A. P., and Gallagher, J. T.,** Mucous glycoproteins: a gel of a problem, *Essays Biochem.,* 20, 40, 1985.
13. **Schachter, H.,** Glycoproteins: their structure, biosynthesis and possible clinical implications, *Clin. Biochem.,* 17, 3, 1984.
14. **Forstner, J. F., Jabbal, I., Qureschi, R., Kells, D. I. C., and Forstner, G. G.,** The role of disulphide bonds in human intestinal mucin, *Biochem. J.,* 181, 725, 1979.
15. **Marshall, T. and Allen, A.,** The isolation and characterization of the high-molecular-weight glycoprotein from pig colonic mucus, *Biochem. J.,* 173, 569, 1978.
16. **Smith, A. C. and Podolsky, D. K.,** Colonic mucus glycoprotein in health and disease, *Clin. Gastroenterol.,* 15, 815, 1986.
17. **Allen, A. and Snary, D.,** The structure and function of gastric mucus, *Gut,* 13, 666, 1972.
18. **Allen, A.,** Structure of gastrointestinal mucus glycoproteins and the viscous and gel-forming properties of mucus, *Br. Med. Bull.,* 34, 28, 1978.
19. **Carlstedt, I. and Sheehan, J. K.,** Macromolecular properties and polymeric structure of mucus glycoproteins, in *Mucus and Mucosa, Ciba Found. Symp. 109,* Pitman Publishing, Marshfield, MA, 1984, 157.
20. **Sheehan, J. K., Oates, K., and Carlstedt, I.,** Electron microscopy of cervical, gastric, and bronchial mucus glycoproteins, *Biochem. J.,* 239, 147, 1986.
21. **Carlstedt, I. and Sheehan, J. K.,** Is the macromolecular architecture of cervical, respiratory and gastric mucins the same?, *Biochem. Soc. Trans.,* 12, 615, 1984.
22. **Mantle, M. and Forstner, J. F.,** The effects of delipidation on the major antigenic determinant of purified human intestinal mucin, *Biochem. Cell Biol.,* 64, 223, 1986.
23. **Slomiany, A., Slomiany, B. L., Witas, H., Aono, M., and Newman, L. J.,** Isolation of fatty acids covalently bound to the gastric mucus glycoprotein of normal and cystic fibrosis patients, *Biochem. Biophys. Res. Commun.,* 113, 286, 1983.
24. **Slomiany, A., Witas, A., Aono, M., and Slomiany, B. L.,** Covalently linked fatty acids in gastric mucus glycoprotein of cystic fibrosis patients, *J. Biol. Chem.,* 258, 8535, 1983.
25. **Slomiany, A., Jozwiak, Z., Takagi, A., and Slomiany, B. L.,** The role of covalently bound fatty acids in the degradation of human gastric mucus glycoprotein, *Arch. Biochem. Biophys.,* 229, 560, 1984.
26. **Marshall, R. D.,** Genetic aspects of glycoproteins, *Biochem. Soc. Trans.,* 12, 513, 1984.
27. **Schacter, H. and Williams, D.,** Biosynthesis of mucus glycoproteins, *Adv. Exp. Med. Biol.,* 144, 3, 1982.
28. **Sharon, N.,** Glycoproteins, *TIBS,* 9, 198, 1984.

29. **LaMont, J. T. and Ventola, A.,** Galactosyltransferase in fetal, neonatal, and adult colon: relationship to differentiation, Part A, *J. Physiol.,* 235, E213, 1978.
30. **Paulsen, H.,** Synthesis of complex oligosaccharide chains of glycoproteins, *Chem. Soc. Rev.,* 13, 15, 1984.
31. **Allen, A., Cunliffe, W. J., Hutton, D. A., and Pearson, J. P.,** Gastrointestinal mucus, *Topics Gastroenterol.,* 12, 211, 1985.
32. **Florey, H.,** The secretion of mucus by the colon, *Br. J. Exp. Pathol.,* 11, 348, 1930.
33. **Florey, H. W.,** The secretion of mucus and inflammation of mucous membranes, in *General Pathology,* Florey, H. W., Ed., Lloyd-Luke, 1970, 195.
34. **Florey, H. W.,** The secretion and function of intestinal mucus, *Br. J. Exp. Pathol.,* 43, 326, 1962.
35. **Basbaum, C.,** Regulation of mucus secretion in the intestine, *Gastroenterol. Clin. Biol.,* 9, 45, 1985.
36. **Specian, R. D. and Neutra, M. R.,** Mechanism of rapid mucus secretion in goblet cells stimulated by acetylcholine, *J. Cell Biol.,* 85, 626, 1980.
37. **Neutra, M. R., O'Malley, L. J., and Specian, R. D.,** Regulation of intestinal goblet cell secretion, II. A survey of potential secretagogues, *Am. J. Physiol.,* 242, G380, 1982.
38. **Neutra, M. R., Phillips, T. L., and Phillips, T. E.,** Regulation of intestinal goblet cells *in situ,* in mucosal explants and in the isolated epithelium, in *Mucus and Mucosa, Ciba Found. Symp.,* 109, Pitman Publishers, Marshfield, MA, 1984, 20.
39. **Smith, B. and Butler, M.,** The autonomic control of colonic mucin secretion in the mouse, *Br. J. Exp. Pathol.,* 55, 615, 1974.
40. **Bradbury, J. E., Black, J. W., and Wyllie, J. H.,** Stimulation of mucus output from rat colon *in vivo, Eur. J. Pharmacol.,* 68, 417, 1980.
41. **Forstner, G., Shih, M., and Lukie, B.,** Cyclic AMP and intestinal glycoprotein synthesis: the effect of beta-adrenergic agents, theophylline, and dibutyryl cyclic AMP, *Can. J. Physiol. Pharmacol.,* 51, 122, 1973.
42. **Roomi, N., Laburthe, M., Fleming, N., Crowther, R., and Forstner, J.,** Cholera-induced mucin secretion from rat intestine: lack of effect of cAMP, cycloheximide, VIP, and cholchicine, *Am. J. Physiol.,* 247, G140, 1984.
43. **Phillips, T. E., Phillips, T. H., and Neutra, M. R.,** Regulation of intestinal goblet cell secretion. III. Isolation intestinal epithelium, *Am. J. Physiol.,* 247, G674, 1984.
44. **Neutra, M. R., Grand, R. J., and Trier, J. S.,** Glycoprotein synthesis, transport, and secretion by epithelial cells of human rectal mucosa, *Lab. Invest.,* 36, 535, 1977.
45. **LaMont, J. T. and Szabo, S.,** Stimulatory effects of prostaglandin and cysteamine on gastric mucus glycoprotein secretion, in *Mechanisms of Mucosal Protection in the Upper GI Tract,* Allen, A., Flemstrom, G., Garner, A., Silen, W., and Turnberg, L. A., Eds., Raven Press, New York, 1984, 241.
46. **Bersimbaev, R. I., Taivov, M. M., and Salganik, R. I.,** Biochemical mechanisms of regulation of mucus secretion by prostaglandin E^2 in rat gastric mucosa, *Eur. J. Pharmacol.,* 115, 259, 1985.
47. **Rainford, K. D.,** The effects of aspirin and other non-steroidal anti-inflammatory drugs on gastrointestinal mucus glycoprotein synthesis *in vivo:* relationship to ulceragenic actions, *Biochem. Pharmacol.,* 27, 877, 1978.
48. **Walker, W. A., Wu, M., and Bloch, K. J.,** Stimulation by immune complexes of mucus release from goblet cells of the rat small intestine, *Science,* 197, 370, 1977.
49. **Lake, A. M., Bloch, K. J., Neutra, M. R., and Walker, W. A.,** Intestinal goblet cell release. II. *In vivo* stimulation by antigen in the immunized rat, *J. Immunol.,* 122, 834, 1979.
50. **Lake, A. M., Bloch, K. J., Sinclair, K. J., and Walker, W. A.,** Anaphylactic release of intestinal goblet cell mucus, *Immunology,* 39, 173, 1980.
51. **Florey, H.,** Mucin and the protection of the body, *Proc. Soc. London Ser. B,* 143, 147, 1955.
52. **Tanaka, T., Sun, S. -T., Hirokawa, Y., Katayama, S., Kucera, J., Hirose, Y., and Amiya, T.,** Mechanical instability of gels at the phase transition, *Nature,* 325, 796, 1987.
53. **Verdugo, P.,** Hydration kinetics of exocytosed mucins in cultured secretory cells of the rabbit trachea: a new model, in *Mucus and Mucosa: Ciba Foundation Symposium 109,* Pitt, London, 1984, 212.
54. **Perman, J. A. and Modler, S.,** Glycoproteins as substrates for production of hydrogen and methane by colonic bacterial flora, *Gastroenterology,* 83, 388, 1982.
55. **Variyam, E. P. and Hoskins, L. C.,** Mucin degradation in human colon ecosystems—degradation of hog gastric mucin by fecal extracts and fecal cultures, *Gastroenterology,* 81, 751, 1981.
56. **Miller, R. S. and Hoskins, L. C.,** Mucin degradation in human colon ecosystems—fecal population densities of mucin-degrading bacteria estimated by a "most probable number" method, *Gastroenterology,* 81, 759, 1981.
57. **Hoskins, L. C. and Zamcheck, N.,** Bacterial degradation of gastrointestinal mucins. I. Comparison of mucus constituents in the stools of germ-free and conventional rats, *Gastroenterology,* 54, 210, 1968.
58. **Prizont, R. and Konigsberg, N.,** Identification of bacterial glycosidases in rat cecal contents, *Dig. Dis. Sci.,* 26, 773, 1981.

59. **Rhodes, J. M., Black, R. R., Gallimore, R., and Savage, A.,** Histochemical demonstration of desialation and desulphation of normal and inflammatory bowel disease rectal mucus by faecal extracts, *Gut,* 26, 1312, 1985.

60. **Stanley, R. A., Ram, S. P., Wilkinson, R. K., and Roberton, A. M.,** Degradation of pig gastric and colonic mucins by bacteria isolated from the pig colon, *Appl. Environ. Microbiol.,* 51, 1104, 1986.

61. **Cook, H. C.,** Carbohydrates, in *Manual of Histological Demonstration Techniques,* Butterworths, London, 1974, 194.

62. **Cook, H. C.,** Carbohydrates, in *Theory and Practice of Histological Techniques,* Bancroft, J. D. and Stevens, A., Eds., Churchill Livingstone, London, 1977, 147.

63. **Filipe, M. I.,** Mucins in the human gastrointestinal epithelium: a review, *Invest. Cell Pathol.,* 2, 195, 1979.

64. **Culling, C. F., Reid, P. A., and Dunn, W. L.,** A histological comparison of O-acetylated sialic acids of the epithelial mucins in ulcerative colitis, Crohn's disease, and normal controls, *J. Clin. Pathol.,* 32, 1272, 1979.

65. **Greco, V., Lauro, G., Fabbrini, A., and Toroli, A.,** Histochemistry of the colonic epithelial mucins in normal subjects and in patients with ulcerative colitis, *Gut,* 8, 491, 1967.

66. **Filipe, M. I.,** Value of histochemical reactions for mucosubstances in the diagnosis of certain pathological conditions of the colon and rectum, *Gut,* 10, 577, 1969.

67. **Reid, P. E., Culling, C. F. A., Dunn, W. L., Ramey, C. W., and Clay, M. G.,** Chemical and histochemical studies of normal and diseased human gastrointestinal tract. I. A comparison between histologically normal colon, colonic tumours, ulcerative colitis and diverticular disease of the colon, *Histochem. J.,* 16, 235, 1984.

68. **Filipe, M. I. and Dawson, I.,** The diagnostic value of mucosubstances in rectal biopsies from patients with ulcerative colitis and Crohn's disease, *Gut,* 11, 229, 1970.

69. **Ehsanullah, M., Filipe, M. I., and Gassard, B.,** Mucin secretion in inflammatory bowel disease: correlation with disease activity and dysplasia, *Gut,* 23, 485, 1982.

70. **Dawson, I. M. P.,** The value of histochemistry in the diagnosis and prognosis of gastrointestinal diseases, in *Histochemistry: The Widening Horizons,* Stoward, P. J. and Polak, J. M., Eds., John Wiley & Son, New York, 1981, 127.

71. **Rogers, C. M., Cooke, K. B., and Filipe, M. I.,** Sialic acids of human large bowel mucosa: O-acylated variants in normal and malignant states, *Gut,* 19, 587, 1985.

72. **Boland, C. R. and Ahnen, D. J.,** Binding of lectins to goblet cell mucin in malignant and premalignant colonic epithelium in the DF-1 mouse, *Gastroenterology,* 89, 127, 1985.

73. **Jacobs, L. R. and Huber, P. W.,** Regional distribution and alterations of lectin binding to colorectal mucin in mucosal biopsies from controls and subjects with inflammatory bowel disease, *J. Clin. Invest.,* 75, 112, 1985.

74. **Machell, R. J. and Stoddart, R. W.,** Rectal goblet cell mucous glycoproteins in ulcerative colitis: studies using fluorescein-labelled lectins, *Gut,* 18, 411, 1977.

75. **Eastwood, G. L. and Trier, J. S.,** Epithelial cell renewal in cultured rectal biopsies in ulcerative colitis, *Gastroenterology,* 64, 383, 1973.

76. **Kanemitsu, T., Koike, A., and Yamamoto, S.,** Study of the cell proliferation kinetics in ulcerative colitis, adenomatous polyps, and cancer, *Cancer,* 56, 1094, 1985.

77. **Franklin, W. A., McDonald, G. B., Stein, H. O., Gatter, K. C., Jewell, D. P., Clarke, L. C., and Mason, D. Y.,** Immunohistologic demonstration of abnormal colonic crypt cell kinetics in ulcerative colitis, *Hum. Pathol.,* 16, 1129, 1985.

78. **Allan, A., Bristol, J. B., and Williamson, R. C. N.,** Crypt cell production rate in ulcerative proctocolitis: differential increments in remission and relapse, *Gut,* 26, 999, 1985.

79. **Shields, H. M., Bates, M. L., Goldman, H., Zuckerman, G. R., Mills, B. A., Best, C. J., Bair, F. A., Goran, D. A., and DeSchryver-Kecskemeti, K.,** Scanning electron microscopic appearances of chronic ulcerative colitis with and without dysplasia, *Gastroenterology,* 89, 62, 1985.

80. **Barton, W., Brown, P., and Clamp, J. R.,** The carbohydrate content of mucosal biopsies, *Clin. Chim. Acta,* 36, 262, 1972.

81. **Fraser, G. M. and Clamp, J. R.,** Changes in human colonic mucus in ulcerative colitis, *Gut,* 16, 832, 1975.

82. **LaMont, J. T. and Ventola, A. S.,** Purification and composition of colonic epithelial mucin, *Biochim. Biophys. Acta,* 626, 234, 1980.

83. **Podolsky, D. K. and Isselbacher, K. J.,** Composition of human colonic mucin—selective alteration in inflammatory bowel disease, *J. Clin. Invest.,* 72, 142, 1983.

84. **Podolsky, D. K. and Isselbacher, K. J.,** Glycoprotein composition of colonic mucosa—specific alterations in ulcerative colitis, *Gastroenterology,* 87, 991, 1984.

85. **Slomiany, B. L., Murty, V. L. N., and Slomiany, A.,** Isolation and characterization of oligosaccharides from rat colonic mucus glycoproteins, *J. Biol. Chem.,* 255, 9719, 1980.

86. **Podolsky, D. K.,** Oligosaccharide structures of human colonic mucin, *J. Biol. Chem.,* 260, 8262, 1985.

87. **Podolsky, D. K., Fournier, D. A., and Lynch, K. E.,** Development of anti-human colonic mucin monoclonal antibodies—characterization of multiple colonic mucin species, *J. Clin. Invest.,* 77, 1251, 1986.

88. **Podolsky, D. K., Fournier, D. A., and Lynch, K. E.,** Human colonic goblet cells—demonstration of distinct populations defined by mucin-specific monoclonal antibodies, *J. Clin. Invest.,* 77, 1263, 1986.

89. **Rhodes, J. M., Parker, N., Patel, P., and Ching, C. K.,** Colonic mucin subclass defect in ulcerative colitis: real or artifact?, *Gut,* 27, A1276, 1986.

90. **McDermott, R. P., Donaldson, R. M., Jr., and Trier, J. S.,** Glycoprotein synthesis and secretion by mucosal biopsies of rabbit colon and human rectum, *J. Clin. Invest.,* 54, 545, 1974.

91. **LaMont, J. T. and Ventola, A.,** Stimulation of colonic glycoprotein synthesis by dibutyryl cyclic AMP and theophylline, *Gastroenterology,* 72, 82, 1977.

92. **Burton, A. F. and Anderson, F. H.,** Decreased incorporation of ^{14}C-glucosamine relative to ^{3}H-N-acetyl glucosamine in the intestinal mucosa of patients with inflammatory bowel disease, *Am. J. Gastroenterol.,* 78, 19, 1983.

93. **Cope, G. F., Heatley, R. V., Kelleher, J., and Axon, A. T. R.,** *In vitro* mucus glycoprotein production by colonic tissue from patients with ulcerative colitis, *Gut,* 29, 229, 1988.

94. **Machell, R. J. and Stoddart, R. W.,** Rectal goblet cell mucous glycoproteins in ulcerative colitis: studies using fluorescein-labelled lectins, *Gut,* 18, 411, 1977.

95. **Smith, A. C. and Podolsky, D. K.,** Biosynthesis and secretion of human colonic mucin glycoproteins, *J. Clin. Invest.,* 80, 300, 1987.

96. **Goodman, M. J., Kent, P. W., and Truelove, S. C.,** Glucosamine synthetase activity in the colonic mucosa in ulcerative colitis and Crohn's disease, *Gut,* 16, 833, 1975.

97. **Rhodes, J. M., Gallimore, R., Elias, E., Allan, R. N., and Kennedy, J. F.,** Faecal mucus degrading glycosidases in ulcerative colitis and Crohn's disease, *Gut,* 26, 761, 1985.

98. **Rhodes, J. M., Gallimore, R., Elias, E., and Kennedy, J. F.,** Faecal sulphatase in health and in inflammatory bowel disease, *Gut,* 26, 466, 1985.

99. **Corfield, A. P., Williams, A. J. K., Wagner, S. A., Clamp, J. R., and Mountford, R. A.,** Mucus glycoprotein degrading enzymes in inflammatory bowel disease detection of a novel sialic acid O-acetyl esterase, *Gut,* 27, A1261, 1986.

100. **Rhodes, J., Gallimore, R., Elias, E., Allan, R., and Kennedy, J.,** Faecal mucus-degrading glycosidases in ulcerative colitis and Crohn's disease, *Clin. Sci.,* 64, 33, 1983.

101. **Hodgson, H. J. K. and Jewell, D. P.,** Immunology of inflammatory bowel disease, *Baillier's Gastroenterol.,* 531, 1987.

102. **Nielsen, O. H., Ahnfelt-Ronne, I., and Elmgreen, J.,** Abnormal metabolism of arachidonic acid in chronic inflammatory bowel disease: enhanced release of leucotriene B^4 from activated neutrophils, *Gut,* 28, 181, 1987.

103. **Rampton, D. S. and Sawkey, C. J.,** Prostaglandins and ulcerative colitis, *Gut,* 25, 1399, 1984.

104. **Sharon, P., Ligumsky, M., Rachmilewitz, D., and Zor, U.,** Role of prostaglandins in ulcerative colitis—enhanced production during active disease and inhibition by sulfasalazine, *Gastroenterology,* 75, 638, 1978.

105. **Sharon, P. and Stenson, W. F.,** Enhanced synthesis of leukotriene B^4 by colonic mucosa in inflammatory bowel disease, *Gastroenterology,* 86, 453, 1984.

106. **Bolton, J. P., Palmer, D., and Cohen, M. M.,** Stimulation of mucus and non-parietal cell secretion by the E^2 prostaglandins, *Dig. Dis.,* 23, 359, 1978.

107. **Harries, A. D., Baird, A., and Rhodes, J.,** Non-smoking: a feature of ulcerative colitis, *Br. Med. J.,* 284, 706, 1982.

108. **Jick, H. and Walker, A. M.,** Cigarette smoking and ulcerative colitis, *N. Engl. J. Med.,* 308, 261, 1983.

109. **Tobin, M. V., Logan, R. F. A., Langman, M. J. S., McConnell, R. B., and Gilmore, I. T.,** Cigarette smoking and inflammatory bowel disease, *Gastroenterology,* 93, 316, 1987.

110. **Cope, G. F., Heatley, R. V., Kelleher, J., and Lee, P. N.,** Cigarette smoking and inflammatory bowel disease: a review, *Hum. Toxicol.,* 6, 189, 1987.

111. **Somerville, K. W., Logan, R. F. A., Edmond, M., and Langman, M. J. S.,** Smoking and Crohn's disease, *Br. Med. J.,* 289, 954, 1984.

112. **De Castella, H.,** Non-smoking: a feature of ulcerative colitis, *Br. Med. J.,* 284, 1706, 1982.

113. **Franceschi, S., Panza, E., La Vecchia, C., Parazzini, F., Decarli, A., and Porro, G. B.,** Non specific inflammatory bowel disease and smoking, *Am. J. Epidemiol.,* 125, 445, 1987.

114. **Lindberg, E., Tysk, C., Andersson, K., and Jarneerot, G.,** Smoking and inflammatory bowel disease. A case-control study, *Gut,* 29, 352, 1988.

115. **Boyko, E. J., Koepell, T. D., Perera, D. R., and Inui, T. S.,** Risk of ulcerative colitis among former and current cigarette smokers, *N. Engl. J. Med.,* 3126, 707, 1987.

116. **Cope, G. F., Heatley, R. V., and Kelleher, J.,** Smoking and colonic mucus in ulcerative colitis, *Br. Med. J.,* 293, 481, 1986.

117. **Cope, G. F., Heatley, R. V., and Kelleher, J.,** Does the cessation of smoking predispose to ulcerative colitis by reducing colonic mucus production?, *Gut,* 29, 704, 1988.

Chapter 8

CHARACTERISTICS OF ANIMAL MODELS OF INFLAMMATORY BOWEL DISEASE

Thérèse McCall and Nigel K. Boughton-Smith

TABLE OF CONTENTS

I. INTRODUCTION

The etiology of ulcerative colitis is poorly understood. Furthermore, the treatment of this disease is far from satisfactory. The understanding of this disease may be increased by the study of animal models of inflammatory bowel disease (IBD).

A variety of experimental animals models of IBD have been developed (Table 1). These models have been used both to gain a greater understanding of the pathophysiology of the disease and to aid in the search for more effective and novel therapies for the treatment of the disease.

None of the induced models of IBD or the spontaneous lesions occurring in various species exactly mimics the human disease. However, many features of these models are similar to aspects of the disease in man and can be used to investigate the role of specific inflammatory processes that may underlie the disease in man or provide a clue as to novel means of therapeutic intervention.

In the present chapter the major approaches to producing animal models of IBD are reviewed. In addition, studies involving animal models and the role of eicosanoids in IBD are described.

II. HAPTEN-INDUCED MODELS OF COLITIS

A. DINITROCHLOROBENZENE

A model of colitis was originally described by Rosenberg and Fischer[1] based on the concept of contact dermatitis. The skin of guinea pigs is painted with a solution of the hapten 1-chloro-2,4-dinitrobenzene (DNCB), and 7 d later, a mixture of DNCB in an adherent dental paste (Orabase®) is instilled intrarectally. After 24 h, histological examination of the colon reveals an allergic reaction consisting of edema, vasodilation, and an intense perivascular accumulation of inflammatory cells, with some migration into the mucosa.[1] The colonic inflammation in animals challenged with 1% DNCB is found to be more consistent than in animals receiving 0.25% DNCB.[2] In control guinea pigs receiving 1% DNCB intrarectally after application of ethanol to the skin or challenged with Orabase® vehicle af er previous sensitization to DNCB, there is no inflammation, indicating the absolute require ent for previous sensitization.

Histological examination of the colons shows mucosa and submucosal inflammatory cell infiltration, mucus depletion from goblet cells, and ucosal edema and hyperemia. By electron microscopy, the inflammatory cell infiltrate is omposed predominantly of lymphocytes, monocytes, and macrophages. There is also an inf tration of neutrophils, basophils, and eosinophils.[3] This model of colitis is unresponsive to antiinflammatory drugs;[2,4] however, whether this is due to the insensitivity of the species used to these drugs or to the disease mechanism is not clear.

B. TRINITROBENZENE SULFONIC ACID

A more recently described model of IBD, induced in rats by the hapten trinitrobenzene sulfonic acid (TNB), has provided a useful tool to expand research into IBD.[5] In this model, a single instillation of TNB into the rat colon produces a chronic ulceration and inflammation. The hapten is dissolved in ethanol and it is assumed that this acts as a "barrier breaker" allowing the hapten access to the lamina propria which then induces a chronic inflammatory response. In this model the colonic damage produced includes open ulceration and skip lesions that persist for at least 5 weeks. The histopathological features have some resemblance to Crohn's disease, in particular the basal lymphoid aggregates, granulomata, and the presence of giant cells.

The morphological and histological changes in the structure of the rat colon following TNB are shown in Figure 1. The normal rat colon has a white, pearly, semitranslucent appearance.

TABLE 1
Animal Models of
Inflammatory Bowel Disease

Immunological
  Hapten induced
  Hypersensitivity reactions
Chemical irritants
  Acetic acid
  Ethanol
Carrageenan (seaweed)
Bacterial infection
  Bacteria
  Antibiotics
Ischemia
  Cholinergic agents
  Mechanical obstruction
Spontaneous lesions

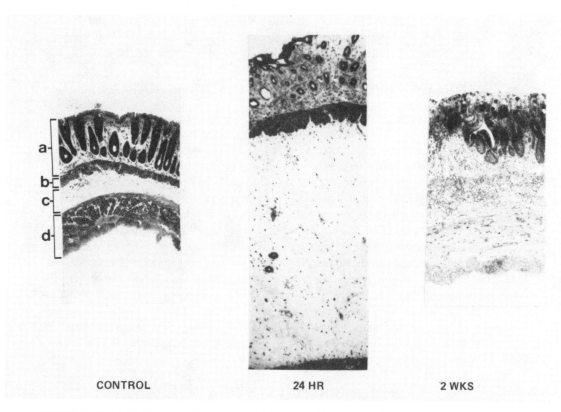

CONTROL   24 HR   2 WKS

FIGURE 1. Histological sections of rat colon showing effects of intracolonic trinitrobenzene sulfonic acid (20 mg, 0.25 ml of 30% ethanol). Indicated on control colon are (a) mucosa, (b) muscularis mucosa, (c) submucosa, and (d) muscularis. There is marked mucosal necrosis, submucosal edema, inflammatory cell infiltration 24 h after TNB. At 2 weeks after TNB, the glands remain disorganized and the marked cellular infiltration persists, there is also some muscle thickening. (Methylene blue-azure II basic fuschia stain, magnification × 80.)

Histologically, the epithelium is intact and the glandular mucosa is organized and filled with mucus. The muscularis mucosa, the submucosa, and the muscularis are clearly delineated. There is necrosis of the mucosa 24 h after TNB and this is accompanied by submucosal edema and cellular infiltration. At 2 weeks after TNB, there is some restitution of the mucosa and a decrease in edema, but the glands remain disorganized and there is a marked cellular infiltrate into all layers of the colon. Muscle thickening is also a feature of this chronic phase of the model.

The development of chronic inflammation in this model can be investigated by measuring changes in the inflammatory cell infiltration into the colon using both histological techniques and the activity of myeloperoxidase (MPO).[6] MPO is a hemoprotein found specifically in phagocytic cells, particularly neutrophils, which catalyzes the peroxidation of a wide variety of substrates and is involved in intracellular bacterial killing. This enzyme has been used as a marker for polymorphonuclear leukocyte infiltration into a wide variety of tissues.

Increases in MPO activity in the chronic phase of this model of IBD were assessed 3 weeks after intrarectal administration of different concentrations of TNB and were directly related to the macroscopic damage of the colon. In addition, increased MPO activity correlates with a decrease in body weight gain (Figure 2), an indication of the general well being of the rats. There are also increases in the colonic formation of the proinflammatory lipid mediator leukotriene B_4 by the inflamed colon in the chronic phase of the TNB model.

III. DIRECT APPLICATION OF CHEMICAL IRRITANTS

Colonic lesions can be produced in rats and cats by direct exposure of the mucosa to chemical irritants such as acetic acid or ethanol. The lesions following topical damage, which heal slowly, may result from impaired vascularization of the mucosa.[7] Intraluminal instillation of acetic acid (5%) into a ligated segment of ascending colon produced an acute inflammatory response in the mucosa and submucosa, as determined 24 h later. The inflammation was characterized histologically by neutrophil infiltration, hemorrhage, edema, and ulceration.

Acute damage to the rat colon can be induced by local application of dilute ethanol administered intrarectally. The damage is characterized as regions of extensive hyperemia and hemorrhage.[8] Histologically, the mucosal surface of the ethanol-treated colons is completely destroyed and there is extensive necrosis of the mucosal tissue. Disruption of mucosal cells can be assessed by measuring the intraluminal release *in vitro* of the cytoplasmic enzyme marker, lactate dehydrogenase, and the lysosomal enzyme, acid phosphatase. In experiments to determine the protective effects of prostaglandins on the colonic mucosa, animals are pretreated with the prostaglandin analogue, 16,16-dimethyl PGE_2. This stable prostaglandin analogue reduced the ethanol-induced colonic hyperemia and hemorrhage and almost completely abolished the colonic release of the cytoplasmic enzyme (Table 2).

IV. HYPERSENSITIVITY REACTIONS

Various models of colitis have been developed by inducing Arthus, Schwartz, Auer, and direct antigen-antibody hypersensitivity reactions in the colon. Kirsner and colleagues originally described a model of colitis induced by a modification of the Auer reaction in which rabbits, sensitized to egg albumin, had dilute formalin instilled into the rectum, followed by i.v. infusion of antigen.[9] Similarly, i.v. infusion of preformed immune complexes of human serum albumin (HSA) and anti-HSA into nonsensitized rabbits, after previous colonic instillation of dilute formalin, also produces a colitis.[10] The colitis induced by most of these immune complex-medicated reactions only lasts a few days although a more chronic colitis can be induced by immunization with common enterobacterial antigen.[11] It is proposed that hypersensitivity to colonic bacterial antigens may be one mechanism whereby an acute colitis becomes chronic.

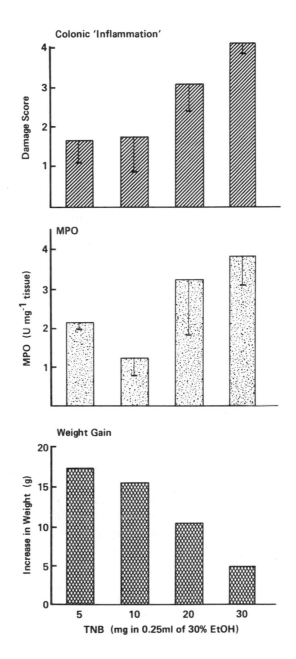

FIGURE 2. The changes in colonic inflammatory (damage score from 0 to 5), myeloperoxidase activity (MPO) and rat weight gain 3 weeks after intracolonic administration of trinitrobenzene sulfonic acid (TNB).

V. CARRAGEENAN-INDUCED COLITIS

Carrageenan is widely used as a food additive. Due to this fact, when Marcus and Watt[12,13] described a novel method for the development of large intestinal ulceration using a 5% aqueous solution of degraded carrageenan, a new field of experimental production of IBD was opened. Carrageenan, a sulfate polysaccharide of high (100,000 to 800,000) molecular weight, is generally extracted from species of red seaweeds, *Chondrus crispus* and *Eucheuma spinosum*. Mild acid hydrolysis results in a degraded material with a molecular weight of 30,000

TABLE 2
Comparative Characteristics of Hapten-Induced Animal Models and
Human Inflammatory Bowel Disease

Parameter	Ulcerative colitis	Crohn's disease	DCNB colitis	TNB colitis
Species	Human	Human	Guinea pig	Rat
Localization	Continuous, rectum—almost always	Discontinuous, rectum—rare, ileum—frequent, perianal	Continuous, rectum—always	Discontinuous, rectum and colon
Gross morphology	Granular texture, mucosal ulceration, loss of haustra, erythemia, bleeding	Fissuring ulcers, edematous mucosa, cobblestone appearance appearance	Diffuse hyperemia, edema, no ulcers, bleeding	Fissuring ulcers, edematous mucosa, bleeding (in acute phase only)
Histology	Mucosal ulceration, distorted crypts, mucus depletion	Transmural ulceration, distorted crypts, fibrosis	No ulceration edema, mucus depletion, hyperemia	Transmural ulceration, distorted crypts, fibrosis common
Leucocytic infiltrate	Mucosa and submucosa, PMN and mononuclear	Transmural, PMN, mononuclear lymphoid aggregates, granuloma, giant cells	Mucosa and submucosa, mononuclear	Transmural PMN and aggregates, lymphoid, granuloma, giant cells
History	Chronic, spontaneous relapse, and remission	Chronic, spontaneous relapse and remission	Heals rapidly without continued challenge	Chronic, heals slowly

but the carrageenan maintains its sulfate content. An aqueous solution of degraded carrageenan, when fed in the drinking water to guinea pigs for 30 d, produces, in all the animals, occult blood in the feces and multiple ulcers in the cecum, colon, and rectum. It is postulated that degraded carrageenan given orally induces damage by a local action on the mucosa rather than by a systemic effect[14] since the carrageenan has no effect on the animals when given parenterally. The possibility that bacterial hydrolysis or other alteration of the carrageenan occurs with release of toxic substances, or that changes in the bacterial flora occur within the colon, cannot be excluded. In fact, the intestinal ulceration induced in guinea pigs by carrageenan is apparently dependent on anaerobic bacteria and can be prevented by metronidazole and clindamycin and does not develop in germ-free rats.[15,16] The ulceration of the bowel, initially observed in guinea pigs, can also be induced in the rat, mouse,[17] Rhesus monkey,[18] and rabbit.[19] In contrast, others have failed to produce ulceration with carrageenan in the rat, hamster, squirrel, monkey, or ferret.[19] The induction of the ulceration is totally dependent on the type and degree of degradation of the carrageenan[17,18] and this phenomenon may explain the variability in the different models studied to date.

VI. BACTERIAL INFECTION

The similarities between ulcerative colitis and the colitis due to infection by specific pathogens has led to investigations into bacterial-induced colitis. Various organisms have been implicated as etiologic for ulcerative colitis; however, to date, investigations have failed to isolate any one specific organism consistently from patients with ulcerative colitis. One possibility is that an organism initiates the disease and then disappears, leaving some process of endogenous activity to perpetuate the chronic inflammation. There is however no direct evidence to support this hypothesis.

Studies on the pathogenesis of diarrhea induced by *Escherichia coli* demonstrate that the enterotoxin produced by *E. coli* can produce a diarrheal syndrome resembling cholera.[21] Injection of dead *E. coli* into the footpad of rats results in diarrhea, bleeding, and ulceration of the colonic mucosa.[22] This effect is prevented by feeding with live *E. coli* and is probably produced by changes in the gut flora. Injection of *E. coli* from patients with ulcerative colitis induces colonic autoantibodies in rabbits but fails to produce histological colitis.[23] In addition, attempts to produce chronic ulcerative colitis with bacteria from infiltrates of feces and rectal mucosa obtained from affected IBD patients have been unsuccessful.[24] The induction of colitis by the injection of colonic extracts in other studies was found to be due to *Salmonella* contamination.[25]

A colitis has been produced in hamsters and guinea pigs by the injection of antibiotics such as clindamycin and penicillin.[26,27] The colitis results from an imbalance of the intestinal flora leading to the release of specific toxins and can be reversed or prevented by administration of antibiotics active against Gram-negative coliform bacteria. This animal model has many of the features of antibiotic-associated colitis in man, but as such does not provide a good model of nonspecific IBD.

VII. VASCULAR IMPAIRMENT

The possibility that ulcerative colitis may have a vascular etiology[28] led to models being induced by restricting blood flow. A bloody diarrhea with histological signs of vascular hyperemia, congestion, and hemorrhage resembling that seen in the early stages of ulcerative colitis in man is produced by the injection of cholinergic agents in dogs.[29] This effect is probably secondary to severe muscular contractions of the bowel wall produced by these drugs and is reversed when drug treatment was stopped. Mucosal ulceration of the dog colon can also be produced by mechanical reduction of colonic blood flow.[30] Marston et al. demonstrated that the healthy colon can withstand ligation of a single major artery. However, ligation of two or more of the major arteries usually results in a circumferential mucosal slough, producing a raw hemorrhagic area of variable size. In this model, mucosal ulceration is directly related to the degree of ischemia inflicted.

VIII. SPONTANEOUS LESIONS

In the search for an authentic model of ulcerative colitis, interest has been directed toward the spontaneous inflammatory lesions of the colon found in some animals. While these lesions have some of the features common to human disease, none have possessed the frequency of occurrence or have had the total characteristic histopathology of ulcerative colitis. The most recently described spontaneous colitis in animals has been in cotton-top tamarins, *Saquinus oedipus*. This colitis is chronic and it responds to sulfasalazine treatment.[31] In this model, acute colitis precedes the spontaneous development of colonic carcinoma following idiopathic ulcerative colitis, which is related to the extent of colonic involvement and the duration of disease, with increased risk per year.

Spontaneous colonic lesions have also been observed in other species including rats, mice, and, in particular, boxer dogs.[32] In boxer dogs, this disease usually begins in puppyhood and has a female:male ratio of 2:1. There is a history of loose, poorly formed stools and the disease is characterized by remissions and exacerbations. An exacerbation may be precipitated by pregnancy and a change in food or environment. Mild to moderate disease has been effectively treated with sulfasalazine. However, in the severe forms of disease, systemic antibiotics and steroids have produced variable results.[32] Genetic predisposition is indicated by the fact that only purebred dogs, after generations of inbreeding and line breeding, possess the disease susceptibilities.[33] As this spontaneously occurring lesion is very rare and cannot be predicted, it is not a suitable investigative model of colitis in man. However, the etiology of this lesion in dogs is unknown and, with continued research, may provide further understanding of the mechanisms underlying the development of the human disease.

IX. THE EICOSANOIDS

The term eicosanoid may be used to describe any 20-carbon fatty acid (eicosa = 20). Since the major C-20 fatty acids formed by mammalian tissues are derived from arachidonic acid (eicosatetraenoic acid), the term eicosanoid is more often used to describe this fatty acid and the family of metabolites formed from it. The liberation of arachidonic acid from phospholipids by the hydrolytic action of phospholipases, particularly phospholipase A_2, is the rate-limiting step in the biosynthesis of the eicosanoids.[34] The metabolism of arachidonic acid occurs by two distinct types of enzyme, cyclooxygenase and lipoxygenase, as shown in Figure 3.

A. CYCLOOXYGENASE METABOLITES

Cyclooxygenase catalyzes the oxidation of arachidonic acid via unstable endoperoxide intermediates, PGG_2 and PGH_2, into the prostaglandins and thromboxane A_2. These prostanoids have potent biological activity on many systems involved in gastrointestinal physiology and pathology. There is considerable evidence to suggest that the vasodilation produced by prostaglandin E_2 (PGE_2) and prostacyclin (PGI_2) is important in the erythema and edema of acute inflammation.[35,36] Inhibition of cyclooxygenase, and therefore prostaglandin formation, by nonsteroidal antiinflammatory drugs is considered to be the mechanism of their antiinflammatory activity.[35-37] The prostaglandins also have a potent effect on intestinal function.[38] The vasodilator prostaglandins increase intestinal blood flow, while PGE_2 and $PGF_{2\alpha}$ stimulate intestinal motility in a variety of species including man. Prostaglandins of the E and F series and their analogues also evoke a watery diarrhea in experimental animals and man, probably mediated by changes in mucosal water and electrolyte secretion.[39,40]

B. LIPOXYGENASE METABOLITES

The major lipoxygenase enzymes are the 12-, 15-, and 5-lipoxygenases, which metabolize arachidonic acid to unstable monohydroperoxy acids (HPETEs) leading to the formation of the more stable monohydroxy acids (HETEs).[37] Further transformation of 5-HPETE leads to the formation of an unstable intermediate leukotriene (LT) A_4, which can be subsequently enzymically transformed to the dihydroxy acid LTB_4 or to the peptido-leukotrienes, LTC_4, LTD_4, and LTE_4.[41]

The lipoxygenase-derived metabolites of arachidonic acid have potent effects in activating leukocytes.[35,36,42] The original finding that 12-HETE was chemotactic for human polymorphonuclear leukocyte has been extended to include the other HETEs and HPETEs. The dihydroxy metabolite, LTB_4, is one of the most potent chemotactic agents known and is a weak inducer of aggregation, lysosomal enzyme release, and superoxide production in polymorphonuclear leukocytes.

C. EICOSANOIDS IN INFLAMMATORY BOWEL DISEASE

Many of the effects of the prostaglandins on the intestine are similar to the clinical manifestations of active IBD.[43] These intestinal actions, combined with the proinflammatory effects of both cyclooxygenase and lipoxygenase products, suggest that metabolites of arachidonic acid may be important in the pathogenesis of IBD.

In order to understand more fully the role of arachidonic acid metabolites, their formation by normal and inflamed animal intestinal tissues taken from a variety of animal models of IBD has been studied by several groups using different experimental techniques. In addition, the

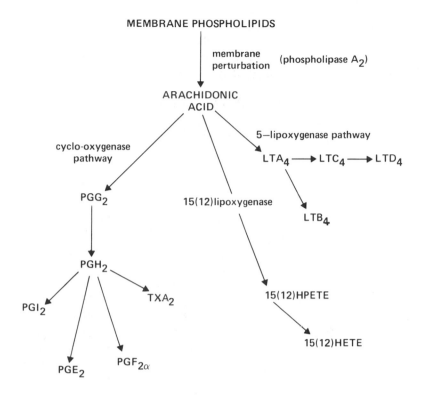

FIGURE 3. Major pathways of arachidonic acid metabolism (PG, prostaglandin; TX, thromboxane; HPETE, hydroperoxyeicosatetraenoic acid; HETE, hydroxyeicosatetraenoic acid; and LT, leukotriene).

effect of antiinflammatory drugs on arachidonic acid metabolism and on the inflammation in colonic tissue from animal models of IBD has also been studied.

D. DNCB MODEL OF COLITIS

Norris et al. originally reported that the level of PGE_2 is elevated in the inflamed colonic mucosa taken from guinea pigs with DNCB colitis.[44] To elucidate further the role of arachidonic acid metabolites, we have investigated the activities of both cyclooxygenase and lipoxygenase enzymes in inflamed colon taken from the DNCB guinea pig model of colitis.[45]

The metabolism of ^{14}C-arachidonic acid by homogenates of inflamed colon taken from guinea pigs with colitis induced by DNCB was substantially increased. There was an increase in the formation of ^{14}C-arachidonic acid metabolites which comigrated with the lipoxygenase products 12- and 15-HETE by inflamed colon. The greatest increase in prostanoid formation was of PGE_2, while there were smaller increases in the formation of PGD_2, TXB_2, $PGF_{2\alpha}$ and 6-keto-$PGF_{1\alpha}$.

The formation of immunoreactive prostanoids from endogenous arachidonic acid was also increased in the inflamed colon.[45] The levels of PGE_2 formed by homogenates of whole colon in our study were similar to those reported in a previous study, using 0.25% DNCB to induce colitis in guinea pigs, that involved the colonic mucosa alone.[44] In that study, blood-free segments of mucosal tissue were frozen in liquid nitrogen before subsequent homogenization. The increases in PGE_2 formation in inflamed colonic mucosa were also similar to our study using whole colon. The formation of TXB_2 and 6-keto $PGF_{1\alpha}$ was also increased in our study on the inflamed guinea pig colon, although under the incubation conditions used, there was no change in immunoreactive LTB_4.[45]

There was also an increase in PGE_2-like activity, measured by bioassay, in homogenates prepared from inflamed large bowel taken from a model of colitis in carrageenin-fed guinea pigs.[46] In addition, microsomes prepared from the inflamed mucosal tissue had an increased capacity to convert ^{14}C-arachidonic acid to radiolabeled PGE_2, while supernatants of the same tissue were found to have a reduced capacity to metabolize $PGF_{2\alpha}$.[46]

E. TNB MODEL OF INFLAMMATORY BOWEL DISEASE

The colonic inflammation induced by TNB was accompanied by increases in colonic myeloperoxidase activity (MPO), an enzymer marker for polymorphonuclear leukocytes.[6] Increases in MPO activity in the acute phase of the TNB model were related to increases in the formation of the lipoxygenase-derived 15-HETE by the inflamed colon as shown in Figure 4. In further studies, the formation of LTB_4 and 6-keto-$PGF_{1\alpha}$ and MPO activity were increased for up to 3 weeks after TNB.[47–49]

The increases in LTB_4 and 6-keto-$PGF_{1\alpha}$ generation by the inflamed rat colon 3 weeks after TNB were reduced to control levels by the experimental antiinflammatory drug BW755C. However, this drug did not consistently reduce the gross ulceration and inflammation.[47] Sulfasalazine and dexamethasone were also without effect in the chronic phase of the TNB model. However, although both these drugs inhibited the increases in 6-keto-$PGF_{1\alpha}$ formation, they had no effect on the formation of LTB_4 by the inflamed colon.[47]

In studies on the acute phase of the TNB model, L651,392, an inhibitor of 5-lipoxygenase, reduced both LTB_4 synthesis and the macroscopic damage but not MPO activity.[48] In the same study, however, BW755C was not effective. In this study only a single dose of each drug was administered into the colon daily and this may not provide a sustained inhibition of lipoxygenase enzymes. Indeed, intracolonic administration of L651,392 did not inhibit LTB_4 synthesis measured 24 h after TNB.[49] The clinically used 5-ASA reduced the colonic damage produced by TNB but was without effect on LTB_4 synthesis or on the levels of MPO in this model.

Treatment with a high dose (20 mg/kg) of 16,16 dimethyl PGE_2 into the colon before TNB reduced the inflammation index, MPO activity, and the production of LTB_4.[50] Furthermore, 16,16 dimethyl PGE_2 treatment after TNB also reduced the inflammation. In another study, pretreatment with a low dose of the prostaglandin analogue rioprostil reduced colonic damage but had no effect on the MPO activity or LTB_4 synthesis.[49] Treatment with rioprostil for 1 week after induction of colitis had no effect.

The beneficial effects of low doses of prostaglandin analogue pretreatment are probably a result of a reduction of the initial colonic injury. However, the beneficial effects of posttreatment with 16,16 dimethyl PGE_2 could be attributed to an antiinflammatory action of this compound which may require higher doses.

F. ACUTE MODELS OF COLITIS

In a model of colitis with damage produced by instillation of acetic acid into the rat colon, there was an increase in arachidonic acid metabolism.[51] Scrapings of inflamed colonic mucosa incubated with ^{14}C-arachidonic acid in the presence or absence of calcium ionophore formed increased levels of radiolabeled metabolites including LTB_4, the lipoxygenase-derived 12- and 15-HETE acids, as well as the cyclooxygenase products. The radiolabeled metabolites were separated by TLC and measured by liquid scintillation counting and unlabeled products were separated by high performance liquid chromatography (HPLC) and measured by UV absorbance.

In rats immunized with the nematode *Nippostronglyus brasiliensis*, i.v. challenge with worm antigen resulted in an anaphylactic response in which the small intestine was the primary shock organ. The subsequent inflammation led to an increase in the luminal release of LTB_4 and LTC_4 and in the level of these leukotrienes in homogenates of gut wall.[52] These events were related to an increase in mucosal mast-cell numbers.

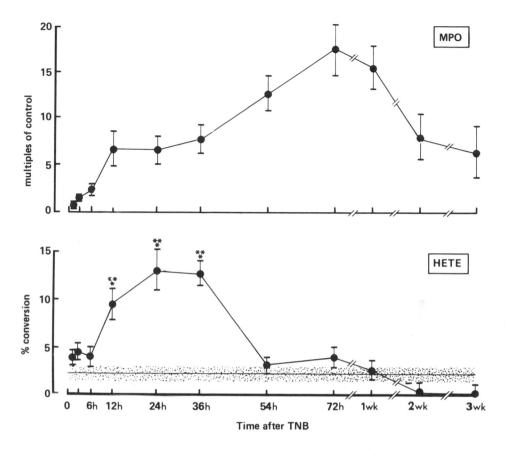

FIGURE 4. Changes in ^{14}C-arachidonic acid (^{14}C-AA) metabolism and myeloperoxidase activity (MPO) in the rat colon following TNB administration. Metabolites of ^{14}C-AA comigrating on TLC with 12/15-HETE (HETE) were formed by homogenates of rat colon and are expressed as percent conversion (percent of total ppm on TLC plate). MPO activity is expressed as multiples of control. The results are the mean ± SEM of (N) rats per group. Control ^{14}C-AA conversion is the mean (single line) and SEM (stippled area of 126 experiments and statistically significant changes are shown by $*$ $p < 0.05$, $**$ $p < 0.01$, and $***$ $p < 0.001$.

In another study, in which chopped colonic tissue from guinea pigs sensitized to ovalbumin was challenged with antigen *in vitro*, there was a considerable release of immunoreactive LTC_4.[53] Separation of the layers of the intestinal wall revealed that the source of immunoreactive LTC_4 was almost exclusively from the colonic mucosa while the formation of 6-keto-$PGF_{1\alpha}$ (which was not increased following ovalbumin challenge) was predominantly from the submucosa.

G. RABBIT MODELS OF COLITIS

An increase in prostanoid formation by vascular-perfused segments of inflamed colon, excised from DNCB or from immune complex-induced colitis in the rabbit, has been reported.[54] The perfused rabbit colons were prelabeled with ^{14}C-arachidonic acid and the prostaglandins and the thromboxane in the venous effluent identified by radiochromatography. Prostanoid formation was also measured by bioassay and immunoassay. The basal formation of PGE_2, TXB_2, and 6-keto-$PGF_{1\alpha}$ by inflamed tissue from both models of colitis was increased. Following bradykinin infusion there was a further increase in prostanoid formation, particularly of TXB_2, which was accompanied by an increase in the vascular perfusion pressure. Angiotensin II also stimulated the formation of PGE_2 and 6-keto-$PGF_{1\alpha}$, but had little effect on TXB_2 synthesis by the rabbit colon.

In further studies on immune complex-induced colitis in the rabbit, eicosanoid release from the rectal mucosa was measured using rectal dialysis.[55] In these studies LTB_4, LTC_4, and PGE_2 were measured by radioimmunoassay, the leukotrienes having been previously separated by HPLC. Eicosanoid formation progressively increased during the development of the inflammation and was correlated with the severity of histologically assessed inflammatory-cell infiltration.

Treatment with methyl prednisolone reduced eicosanoid levels in rectal dialysates; however, they remained considerably higher than in control rabbits.[55] Furthermore, methyl prednisolone had only a minimal effect in the colonic inflammation. Thus, in this model of colitis, steroid therapy was a poor inhibitor of both leukotriene formation and the colitis.

X. DISCUSSION

A variety of animal models of IBD have been developed in a number of different species. These models have been used both to investigate the factors involved in the etiology of the disease and to study the process underlying the intestinal inflammation.

There is no model of IBD that completely mimics the human disease. The present models of IBD do, however, share some characteristics of the disease and provide a means to investigate the role of specific inflammatory mediators and cells in intestinal inflammation.

The possible importance of the metabolites of arachidonic acid in the inflammatory process has led to research into these mediators using animal models of IBD. In various models of IBD, in the guinea pig, rat, and rabbit, increases in the formation of both cyclooxygenase and lipoxygenase metabolites of arachidonic acid have been detected. The increases in eicosanoid formation are usually associated with increases in inflammatory-cell infiltration and the cells composing these infiltrates are a probable source of the lipoxygenase products. Resident leukocytes or other intestinal cells may, however, contribute to the increases in eicosanoid formation. Future studies concerning the contribution of the different cell types to the increase in eicosanoid formation, and the interaction between these cells, will enhance our understanding of the disease process in IBD.

The close association between the increased formation of the potent chemotactic eicosanoid LTB_4 and neutrophil infiltration into the colon is similar to clinical observations in which active colitis is associated with increased formation of both prostaglandins and the leukotrienes. The increases in colonic LTB_4 formation may therefore mediate the pronounced cellular infiltration that is a feature of both active colitis in man and in the animal models of the disease.

Studies with antiinflammatory drugs in models of IBD have given variable effects. The poor response of animal models of IBD may reflect species differences in the sensitivity to antiinflammatory drugs. The severe inflammation and tissue damage in some of the models may require higher doses or a longer duration of drug treatment. Alternatively, the initiation of the tissue damage or the mechanisms underlying the inflammatory response in the models may not be responsive to clinically used drugs such as corticosteroids. Until some of these problems can be resolved, the use of these models for selection of novel therapeutic agents should be viewed with caution.

The increases in colonic LTB_4 formation observed in the models of colitis can be used to determine the bioavailability and potency of novel 5-lipoxygenase inhibitors. These studies will allow the selection of potent, selective, and bioavailable 5-lipoxygenase inhibitors for clinical evaluation in patients with IBD.

Animal models of IBD provide a means of studying the complex process involved in intestinal inflammation and these studies may, in the future, lead to a greater understanding of IBD. These studies will hopefully lead to the development of novel and effective therapies for the treatment of the disease.